The Complete Stretching Book

Look for these books of interest from Runner's World and Collier Books

The Complete Stretching Book

PAUL URAM

COLLIER BOOKS
Macmillan Publishing Company
New York

COLLIER MACMILLAN PUBLISHERS
London

Macmillan Publishing Company
866 Third Avenue, New York, N.Y. 10022
Collier Macmillan Canada, Inc.

Library of Congress Cataloging in Publication Data
Uram, Paul, 1926–
    The complete stretching book.
    1. Exercise.   2. Muscle strength.   3. Stretch
(Physiology)   I. Title.
GV505.U7   1980b   613.7'1   84-16998
ISBN 0-02-029480-8

Macmillan Books are available at special discounts for
bulk purchases for sales promotions, premiums, fund-raising,
or educational use. Special editions or book excerpts
can also be created to specification. For details, contact:
        Special Sales Director
        Macmillan Publishing Company
        866 Third Avenue
        New York, New York 10022

10 9 8 7 6 5 4 3 2 1

Printed in the United States of America

ISBN 0-02-029480-8

I would like to dedicate my efforts to my wife Helen and son Ron, and also to the betterment of athletics.

Contents

Foreword

The Complete Stretching Book summarizes Paul Uram's many years of experience in preparing athletes for competition. Emphasis is placed on the range of motion of joints, their supportive tissues, and musculature. In the past, this aspect of conditioning has been rendered lip service, but most training programs have expended little effort to actually develop it.

Uram's book contains a well-conceived and clearly described program designed to develop maximum range of motion and elasticity of the soft parts of the musculo-skeletal system. It applies to most training programs presently in use throughout the nation, regardless of the specific sport.

Personal experience with his program has shown a decreased incidence of minor muscle pulls and strains which are so aggravating to coaches, trainers, and team physicians. Although statistical verification of this impression is not available, numerous coaches whom I have interviewed strongly support Mr. Uram's program.

We feel that *The Complete Stretching Book* presents a training program that will make competitive athletics a more enjoyable experience for all participants.

James H. McMaster, M.D.
Assistant Professor of Orthopedic Surgery

Peter E. Sheptak, M.D.
Clinical Associate of Neurosurgery

Acknowledgments

This book is the result of many long discussions and general work sessions with my former student Dave McKinnis, who helped with compilation, editing, illustrations, and organization of the material.

Introduction

The programs and ideas presented in this book represent the efforts and observations of my twenty years in athletics. Much of this work is simply a statement of reaffirmation for exercises long known to physical educators and coaches. I have, however, attempted to give some order and reason to the material.

In a time when so many areas of our culture, including athletics, are being severely criticized, I believe it is imperative for teachers and coaches to provide programs of maximum value to the individual. These programs must refine human movement, improve skills, reduce injuries, and, most importantly, promote *lifelong* freedom of movement, thereby restoring a natural attribute that man's mechanized, affluent society has stolen from him.

It is the function of sport to remind man that the human body is the basic tool for life.

After years of applying these exercises and movement patterns to high school gymnasts and professional football players, I am convinced there are definite techniques that refine human movement and that can help everyone realize his or her potential as a complete athlete.

GENERAL PHYSICAL FITNESS

Physical fitness does not describe a state of health but rather a measurement of your efficiency in performing your normal life tasks. Your fitness is determined by genetic structure and by the many environmental factors that affect you, most notably nutrition, rest, exercise, and stress. With proper medical guidance throughout your life you can develop and maintain relatively high levels of general fitness.

A closer look at general physical fitness reveals three distinct areas for development and maintenance. These areas are physique, organic functioning, and muscle responsiveness. *Physique* refers to bone, muscle, and fat proportions. *Organic functioning* refers to cardiovascular and respiratory efficiency as well as the functioning of other major organs such as the kidneys. *Muscle responsiveness*, the third area of general physical fitness, and the major concern of this book, deals with the actions of skeletal or voluntary muscles.

MUSCLE RESPONSIVENESS

Muscle responsiveness has four components: flexibility, strength, speed, and endurance. Flexibility is the suppleness or elasticity of a muscle and its capability to stretch far enough to permit the joint on which it acts to have complete, normal range of motion without injury. Strength, the contractile capacity of the muscle, is the muscle's capability to first move itself through its full range of motion, and to repeat that action against resistance as close to its maximum stress tolerance as possible. Speed is the skill of applying quick contraction to a muscle through its entire range of motion or a specific portion of that range, whether against minimum or maximum resistance. Endurance is the stress tolerance of a muscle as measured by the time a muscle can maintain performance of a specific workload.

An Approach to Developing Muscle Responsiveness

All refined human movement results from some intricate blend of these four muscle responsiveness components. They can never be completely separated. However, refined human movement is best developed by paying attention to the muscle responsiveness components in their most logical order:

1. Developing maximum range of motion first with flexibility exercises, closely followed by (and often accompanied by) strength exercises applied to the full range of motion.

2. Without discarding the flexibility and strength exercises, add speed exercises. The first speed exercises are in the form of full range of motion basic movement patterns.

3. Add progressive overloads to these basic exercises before they are finally applied to a specific skill.

4. Again, without discarding the flexibility, strength, and speed exercises, add endurance exercises. Endurance exercises, like speed exercises, should be applied first to full range of motion basic movement patterns with progressive overloads, and then to developing specific skill endurance.

When all the muscles that act on a joint have reached high levels of muscle responsiveness, the joint will move freely and efficiently through its natural range of motion. Flexibility, strength, speed, and endurance will all be available to any specific skill movement pattern.

Proper development of muscle responsiveness produces additional benefits beyond efficient natural movement. A muscle will show improved tone, efficiency in both contraction and relaxation, an improved blood flow in the capillary network, greater resistance to fatigue, more effective waste product removal, and greater tolerance of stress types that formerly caused injury. An exercise program that pays attention to the concept of muscle responsiveness with progressive flexibility, strength, speed, and endurance exercises also yields wider varieties of movement, improved coordination, agility, balance, quickness, explosiveness, finesse, and, ultimately, refined movement. A well-disciplined exercise program for muscular responsiveness enhances concentration. This in turn facilitates motor learning.

Even though there are many intricate and inseparable relationships among its four components, muscle responsiveness is best developed in a step-like fashion from the simplest and most important level of flexibility to the final and most exhausting level of endurance. The muscle sets must first become sufficiently flexible to permit the joints on which they act to have full and natural range of motion.

A proper flexibility program does not weaken the muscle but actually maintains and improves strength. It also aids the muscle in making greater gains from the strength exercise. When strength exercises are added to the program, the joint will develop more forceful, controlled, natural movement in the newly discovered range of motion. This flexibility-strength phase of the exercise program is the critical first step toward muscle responsiveness for it yields powerful, unrestricted full-range movement.

Speed exercises enter the program next. Their objective is to develop sufficient neuromuscular coordination to build the skill of quick muscular contraction from one length to another and, more importantly, from maximum extension to maximum flexion. The speed exercises won't improve the individual's hereditary gifts but they will lead you to your potential for both quickness and speed.

The final part of the program involves endurance exercises for specific times or until exhaustion, defined here as the inability to perform the movement in a fluid and proper manner. (Exhaustive endurance exercise has meant continuing performance until fatigue prevents further movement, but this is not advocated in this text.)

In the progressive development of muscle responsiveness, the exercises applied to each phase involve only the weight of the related body parts or the weight of the body itself, and only the effort that you can muster unassisted by a partner or device. After developing this free level of muscle responsiveness you can start an overload program of either partner-assisted or device-assisted exercises, or both. The key here is to go through the proper sequence of flexibility, strength, speed, and endurance exercises with the same resistance before moving to a higher degree of overload. As the degree of overload progresses, the need for increased attention to cardiovascular exercise and flexibility also increases. Warmup and warmdown programs that are exclusively designed to step up circulation and stretch all the muscles are imperative.

Principles of Training

A serious and dedicated training program is necessary for the individual to develop a high degree of muscle responsiveness. In addition to using the correct exercise sequence for muscle responsiveness (flexibility, strength, speed, and endurance), you should also observe the following general principles of training:

Readiness. Physical readiness begins when you present clear goals to your coach, trainer, and doctor, and then receive clearance to begin the specific program to attain these goals. Psychological readiness begins when the individual, coach, trainer, and doctor fully understand the goals in sight, the training program and its ordeals, and the emotional stress that may be involved. You are psychologically prepared only when you understand the work and frustrations that are ahead and, through intrinsic motivation, commit yourself to that course of action.

Specificity. Exercises develop the specific muscles that they activate and have their greatest effect on specific areas of these muscles. Specific types of exercise produce specific training benefits: Flexibility exercises produce flexibility, strength exercises produce strength, speed exercises produce speed, endurance exercises produce endurance, and skill exercises produce skill. However, the complex nature of the human body also protects neuromuscular activity in such a way that flexibility exercises may benefit strength maintenance and even strength gains, or strength exercises may benefit flexibility, speed, and endurance. Indeed, the four components of muscle responsiveness are so intricately related that they may all benefit each other. They may also have negative effects on each other, so therefore the underlying principle within the principle of specificity is this: any specific degree of muscle responsiveness must be developed by applying a commensurate specific degree of exercise from all four components—flexibility, strength, speed, and endurance.

Regularity. Exercises should be performed on a regular basis starting and ending at the same times each session. This produces maximum physical and psychological benefit for it allows you to get proper rest and also to anticipate and prepare for the next session. Exercise programs may schedule sessions once each day, many times each day, or once every other day. There are as many possibilities as there are individuals and individual goals, but it is very important to keep the program regular and consistent.

Frequency. How often should you exercise? The answer to this question depends on the intensity of the workload and your response to that workload. Excessive muscular soreness, extreme fatigue, and sudden inappropriate psychological readiness are strong indications that the frequency of the exercise sessions should be reduced, assuming that the individual performs well in the exercise session but simply needs more recovery time afterwards.

In general, low-intensity training in any of the four muscle responsiveness components may be performed each day or several times each day without harm. As the intensity increases and overloads become greater, the rest periods between sessions must be examined and changed when necessary. You and your coach must set specific goals and specific workout times and then train regularly until those goals are reached. The individual may then elect to maintain status quo or establish a new set of goals and a new pattern of regularity.

Adaptation. You go through a process of adjusting and conditioning your level of physical efficiency to meet the new demands of your present exercise program. It is not uncommon in any stage of training, especially in the early stages, to regress in performance. The key here is to be persistent and ride out the storm. Occasionally, it may be advisable to get more rest, or go back and review the fundamentals of a lower intensity training program. But usually if you recognize regression as a natural phenomenon of training, you can continue your workout schedule and pass comfortably through the problem.

Reaching a plateau or leveling off performance for a time is also another natural phenomenon of training and learning. It should be treated in the same way as regression.

Progression, the desirable stage of adaptation, is the step-by-step improvement toward the goals of the training level. The important thing about progression is not to rush but rather to pursue goals in an orderly fashion and attain them degree by degree.

Muscle soreness, fatigue, and psychological frustration are also a natural adaptation of new training levels. For example, soreness may even result from flexibility exercises that normally help reduce soreness. The first stages of any new exercise program are stressful and may make you uncomfortable. Soon, however, your muscles will adapt, the soreness will disappear, and training benefits will begin.

Time of adaptation in any of its forms depends on the individual's unique response to exercise.

Overload. Stepping up the stress intensity of an exercise program to promote a higher level of muscular adaptation is called *overload.* Increased intensity comes from the four R's of exercise—resistance, repetition, rate, and rest. *Resistance,* the force or weight that muscular contraction tries to overcome, may be simply the weight of the related body part, or it may be the weight of a portion of the body or even the entire body weight. Greater resistance comes from gravitational or leverage disadvantages or heavy weights. Strength is measured by the amount of weight a muscle can overcome. Resistance exercises may also be used to promote gains in flexibility, speed, and endurance.

Repetition is the number of times a well-defined exercise is performed correctly. Increases in the number of repetitions of a specific exercise generally produce increases in the specific desired outcomes, at least up to a point of diminishing returns. Repetition has other functions as well: flexibility exercises may be repeated simply to gain additional warmup or warmdown benefits, or to maintain muscular suppleness; repetition of strength, speed, or endurance exercises may also be done simply for maintenance.

Rate is the number of repetitions per unit time. Rate is generally designed to increase stress tolerance and endurance. For example, three repetitions of a ten-second static flexibility exercise performed at random during the day would not have the same beneficial effect of performing those same three repetitions within a one-minute time limit. That change in rate increases intensity, improves stress tolerance, and produces greater flexibility gains.

Rest is the time period between exercise sessions. Rest is also the time period between repetitions of a specific exercise or one set of a specific exercise and one set of another specific exercise. Finally, rest is the quality of relaxation and the effectiveness of recovery from fatigue between exercise sessions or repetitions or sets.

The combination of rate and rest into clearly defined periods of performance and recovery is the basis for interval training. The objective of interval training is to progressively increase the number of repetitions of an exercise within a specific time, decreasing the rest period. These shorter rest periods come as the body develops greater resistance to fatigue. Continued improvement comes when you return to the original intervals and repeat the process with greater resistance providing the overload.

No matter how the four R's of exercise are combined to produce overload, the important thing to remember is that some type of overload is necessary to improve performance.

Measurement. Whether done by sophisticated devices or by simple charts documenting performance improvements, any accurate measurement is valuable to the individual, coach, trainer, or doctor in some way. The value may be purely motivational or it may reveal beneficial and/or detrimental patterns present in the training program.

Warmup and warmdown. Warmups are an essential series of exercises designed to step up circulation, progressively stretch the muscles, improve freedom of motion, and prepare the body for the more vigorous demands of the practice session. They have the additional benefits of promoting relaxation, increasing self-awareness of muscular needs in preparation for an exercise session, and reducing as much as possible the potential for pulls and strains.

Warmdowns are a short series of exercises designed to maintain a slight circulation increase and utilize body warmth (hence the name warmdowns), so that the muscles may benefit from flexibility exercises. These flexibility exercises serve as an additional effort to improve flexibility, but their main objective is to stretch and relax the muscles and promote some immediate removal of fatigue products. Warmdowns aid in reducing muscle soreness that may follow any workout. Warmdowns also increase self-awareness of muscular needs after an exercise session and aid in injury reduction.

Part One

Progressive Development of Muscle Responsiveness

1

Flexibility Training

In modern exercise programs the emphasis is too often on strength, speed, and endurance while flexibility is all but ignored. When flexibility exercises are used, they are often relegated to short warmup programs usually five to seven minutes long. Coaches and trainers tell athletes simply to stretch a little to avoid hamstring or groin pulls. If the short warmup program is well organized and the athletes perform the exercises properly, some warmup benefits result. However, the effects are temporary and yield little or no gains in range of motion, suppleness, resiliency, relaxation, or any of the other benefits of flexibility exercise. The end result is still overemphasis on strength, speed, and endurance.

Exercise and athletic training programs without adequate consideration for flexibility development tend to restrict normal ranges of motion and limit muscle responsiveness. Movement may become awkward and jerky in varying degrees. The athlete may have difficulty in being consistently fluid in the performance of his skills. He or she may become increasingly prone to minor pulls or even serious soft tissue injuries that cause lost training time. He may ultimately limit his skills and training methods to only those activities he knows best and is least afraid to perform. If he is talented and lucky, he may be able to get away with this, but he has sacrificed improvement. He may also have shortened his career.

Lack of flexibility training often produces overtense muscles and disturbs the important neuromuscular function of reciprocal inhibition. Prime-mover muscles or "agonists" tend to shorten too fast while their antagonistic muscles fail to relax easily and completely. This is one important cause of pulls. Another is when overtense helper or synergistic muscles over-stabilize a joint and restrict free movement.

Tight muscles also cause pressure on the capillaries and shunt the blood flow. This prevents oxygen from reaching all the cells properly thus limiting performance, especially endurance tasks. The system also becomes inefficient in carrying away fatigue products. This again limits performance and promotes muscle soreness after performance. Further limitations occur in the areas of relaxation and rest. All these factors make the muscle more injury prone. The muscle is simply working at a disadvantage and inhibiting both the performance and progress of the athlete.

Flexibility exercises are a critical phase of athletic training and the basis for quality muscle responsiveness. Flexibility exercises work to restore normal ranges of motion, improve suppleness and resiliency, promote more efficient blood flow in the capillary network, encourage relaxation, and reduce injury potential in the soft tissues. Additional benefits of improved flexibility include:

1. Proper application of strength, speed, and endurance exercises through the whole range of motion.

2. Greater gains in strength, speed, and endurance.

3. Improved ability to practice and therefore learn a skill.

4. Greater efficiency in skill performance.

5. Improvements in coordination, agility, quickness, balance, and kinesthetic proficiency (thus increasing perceived stimuli and therefore insight into the nature of the skill).

Flexibility exercises in proper combination with strength, speed, and endurance exercises will not reduce joint stability nor weaken muscles, harm tendons, ligaments, or cartilage. It is of course possible to cause damage from abuse of flexibility exercises, just as it is possible to cause damage from any form of exercise. Remember that the development of muscle responsiveness depends on a complete exercise program involving balance of all four components.

Normal flexibility means a muscle can move through its entire length easily and efficiently. When all muscles acting on a joint are flexible, the joint can move through its complete natural range of movement. While that movement is approximately the same for all of us, it is individualized by your specific anatomical structure and by developed structural limitations. The latter include any pathology of the muscles and soft tissues or of the skeletal system.

TYPES OF FLEXIBILITY EXERCISES

There are three basic categories of flexibility exercises. They are rhythmic exercises, static exercises, and resistive exercises.

Rhythmic exercises are simple swinging and rotational movement patterns designed to promote freedom and smoothness of motion. Rhythmic exercises are generally not strenuous and not designed to produce great increases in range of motion. Traditional exercise programs make use of rhythmic flexibility exercises in their simplest form. Examples include arm circles, leg swings, neck and hip rotations. These exercises simply promote relaxation, stimulate circulation, and serve as a mild warmup.

Dance makes the most effective use of rhythmic flexibility exercises. Dancers train for hours repeating complex swinging and rotational movements, and they actually gain in flexibility as well as fluid-controlled movement done in a relaxed manner and with good form. While rhythmic flexibility exercises are of enormous value to the athlete, they are time-consuming and daily progress is slow.

Rhythmics are excellent for athletic specialists (place kickers and punters, pitchers) and these athletes often have time during the week to do rhythmic exercises. For those athletes who do not have time during daily season training, rhythmics make a great off-season form of exercise. They are relatively easy, relaxing, and a positive aid to maintaining freedom of motion without causing injury.

Static flexibility exercises are holds (staying in a given position for a given length of time). Static flexibility exercises can be done alone without special exercise devices. They make effective use of time, and they produce desirable results. Statics also permit the individual to work at his own rate, individualize his efforts to meet his special needs, receive all the benefits of flexibility exercises, and not spend the excessive amounts of time required by rhythmics. You simply select an exercise to stretch a specific area, learn how to perform it properly, and then, using the principles of exercise, set out to make progress toward your goal. Here are some guidelines for best use of static flexibility exercises:

1. Perform the exercise properly to the best of your ability but do not force the muscles to do more than they are ready for or to progress too rapidly.

2. When stretching one set of muscles, also stretch the opposing set. For example, when stretching the hamstring muscles, make sure you also stretch the quadricep muscles.

3. If one set of muscles is particularly tight and needs special attention, stretch the opposing set first. For example, if the hamstrings are tight, stretch the quadriceps first. You will find that the hamstrings respond better to the exercises.

4. Use a complete stretching program rather than limiting your work to one area. You may spend more time on special needs but do it within the context of a complete program. The functioning of one muscle group is almost always related to the functioning of another. For example, special attention to back exercises usually improves the response of both leg and shoulder exercises.

5. Always precede your flexibility workout with brisk walking, jogging, rope skipping, or simple calisthenics to stimulate the circulation. Increased circulation produces greater results from flexibility exercises. Heart rate should be stepped up to at least 100 beats per minute before starting flexibility exercises. It may also be necessary to repeat the procedure several times during the flexibility exercises if your work is slow and permits the heart rate to fall.

6. Keep warm while stretching. Dress in warm clothing and work in a warm gym whenever possible. Warmth enhances all the benefits of flexibility exercises.

7. Learn to recognize stretch pain and use it to your advantage. Stretch pain is the tension, discomfort, and sometimes actual pain that accompanies stretching exercises. Recognize it as a form of feedback from your body and learn to use it properly. In your mind formulate a subjective stretch pain tolerance scale from zero to ten, with ten being your maximum pain tolerance level. When you first begin a stretching program, operate at low stretch pain tolerance levels. After you have exercised several days begin to increase the intensity of your effort and operate at mid-range stretch pain tolerance levels. Finally, after your muscles have adapted to the exercise program, operate on higher and higher levels of stretch pain tolerance. Use this same type of stretch pain tolerance progression in each exercise session, starting at low levels and finishing at higher levels.

At all times pay attention to the kinds of stretch pain that you feel, and identify both the normal and abnormal. Identifying pain will put you more closely in touch with the needs of your muscles. You will soon learn to recognize tensions that are normal and safe, pains that can be relaxed away, pains that can be exercised away, and pains that need rest or special treatment. As you improve your understanding of stretch pain you will be surprised in your ability to: (a) make definite progress in flexibility by doing stretching exercises you once feared; (b) relax away pains which once inhibited you from proper exercise; (c) exercise away pains which you once thought were injuries; (d) recognize symptoms of potential injury you once overlooked; (e) prevent injuries before they happen; and (f) improve your progress in injury therapy.

8. Learn to relax while stretching. Don't hold your breath; breathe normally. Don't fight the exercise; relax your way through it. Don't be frightened by harmless levels of stretch pain and quit; relax away the pain and go on with the exercise. Concentrate and develop your ability to relax while performing a physical task. This type of relaxation promotes great gains in the benefits of exercise.

9. Hold for short periods of time at first and then progress to longer hold times. A beginning static flexibility program should have hold times of three seconds with several repetitions of the exercise. As you adapt to the exercises, increase the hold time to five, then seven seconds, and increase the number of repetitions of the exercise. It is not necessary to hold an exercise for ten seconds or longer. Long holds are beneficial only for special needs. It is much better to hold for five to seven seconds, rest that area while working on another, and then come back to the first area. Hold for short periods of time; use several repetitions; perform the same exercise in standing, seated, and prone positions; keep the exercise program moving, balanced, and interesting.

10. Concentrate on your work. Don't let external or internal disturbances break your concentration. Pay attention to what you are doing. Learn about your muscular need from your body's feedback mechanisms. (Become an expert at focusing your attention on the task at hand.) Strive to increase your self-discipline and your self-knowledge. Make progress.

11. Do not bounce the exercises. Bouncing does not allow the muscle time to sustain the stretched length and benefit from it. Bouncing activates the stretch reflex, thus causing the muscle to contract rather than adapt to the stretched length. This promotes shortening rather than lengthening of the muscle. Bouncing is also dangerous, for it may cause injury.

Resistive flexibility exercises are performed against varying degrees of mild resistance, usually supplied by a partner or some simple device such as a length of surgical tubing. Resistive flexibility exercises not only improve flexibility but also produce moderate strength gains. Resistives are probably the most effective form of flexibility exercise. However, they require time, total cooperation and understanding by the partners, and complete concentration, dedication, and self-discipline. For these reasons they are seldom used successfully. Here are some guidelines for the best use of resistive flexibility exercises:

1. Choose a partner of similar size and strength who has similar needs, and who also has the character and interest to make the program successful for both of you.

2. Perform the exercise properly to the best of your ability but do not force the muscle sets to do more than they are ready for, or to make progress too rapidly.

3. Use the complete stretching program rather than limiting your work to one area. Spend more time on special needs but do it within the context of the entire program.

4. Keep warm while stretching. Dress in warm clothing and work in a warm gym whenever possible.

5. Always stimulate the circulation before starting the program.

6. Learn to relax while exercising. Don't strain or force the exercises. Remember: These exercises are not meant to be a test of strength.

7. Perform the exercise smoothly and do not jerk or snap the movement at any time. The movement should be smooth with constant tension from beginning to end. Reduce the resistance if you cannot perform the exercise properly.

8. Start with short ranges of motion at the relaxed end of the range and with each repetition progress by degrees toward the tighter area.

9. Start with low-range stretch pain tolerance and increase slowly.

10. Start with low resistance and increase slowly to higher levels of resistance. Do not strive for maximum resistance.

11. Always press away from the pain rather than into it. Never force a muscle into the pain area.

12. Concentrate on your work. Pay attention to what you are doing, learn from it, and make progress.

Rhythmic Flexibility Exercises

Stimulate Circulation

Brisk walking, cycling, jogging, or rope skipping for 1 to 5 minutes. Increase the heart rate to over 100 beats per minute.

Arm, Hand, and Shoulder Exercises

Interlock fingers and rotate the wrists in a variety of directions (15 seconds).

(a) Keeping the fingers interlocked, turn the palms *away* from the body, straighten the arms, and:

(b) Swing the arms overhead as high as possible and then swing them back down. Repeat this action in a smooth, even rhythm for ten repetitions.

(c) Extend the arms straight in front of the body and parallel to the floor. Swing from side to side, permitting only the lead arm to bend during the swing.

(d) Extend the arms straight overhead and swing as far as possible from side to side. Swing from the shoulders and upper back.

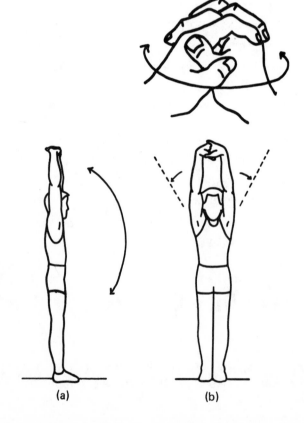

(a)   (b)   (c)

Rhythmic Arm Swings

(a) Forward arm circles—10 repetitions.
(b) Backward arm circles—10 repetitions.
(c) Lateral and vertical arm swings—10 repetitions.
(d) Over-and-under horizontal arm swings—10 repetitions.
(e) Horizontal cross-and-swing—10 repetitions.

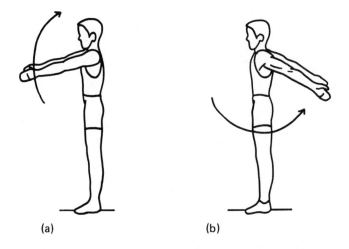

(a)   (b)

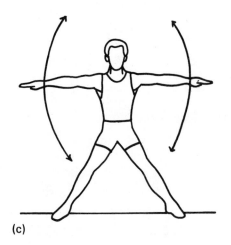

(c)

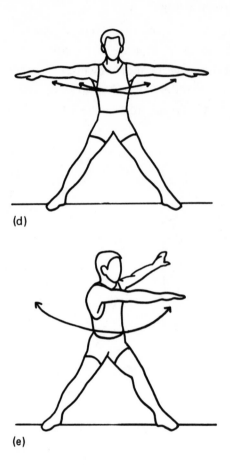

(d)

(e)

Rhythmic Neck Exercises

(a) Move the head side to side laterally, touching right ear to right shoulder, then left ear to left shoulder—10 repetitions.

(b) Move the head forward and backward—10 repetitions.

(c) Turn the head pivotally from side to side—10 repetitions.

(d) Rotate the head in lateral circles right and left—5 repetitions each direction.

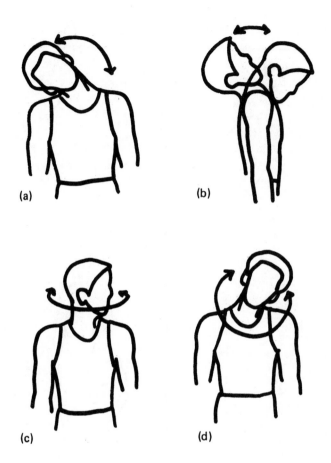

(a)

(b)

(c)

(d)

Rhythmic Trunk Exercises

(a) Place hands on hips and perform simple side bends, alternating sides—5 repetitions each side.

(b) Place hands over head, palms together, arms straight, and repeat the side bends, again alternating sides—5 repetitions each side.

(c) Place hands on hips and perform trunk circles—5 repetitions each side.

(d) Place hands over head, palms together, arms straight, and repeat the trunk circles—5 repetitions each side.

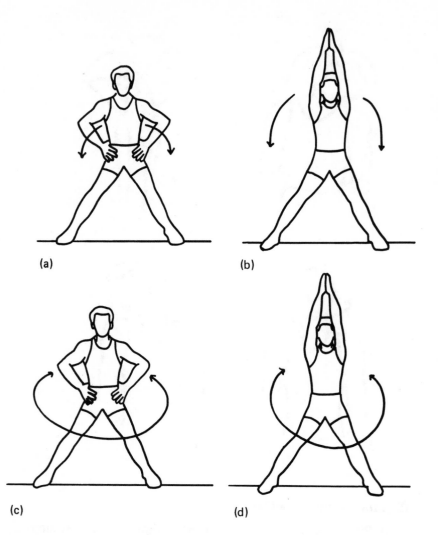

(a)

(b)

(c)

(d)

Rhythmic Body Exercises

(a) *Body wave with legs together.* Swing arms upward and overhead and arch the body. Swing arms back down and round the back, bend at the hips, bend at the knees, and finish the arm swing—10 repetitions.

(b) *Body wave with legs straddled.* Straddle stand with legs just wider than shoulder width. Repeat the body wave as described in (a)—10 repetitions.

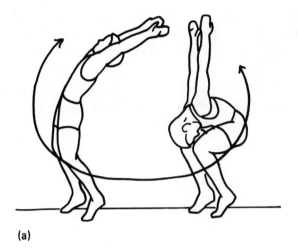

(a)

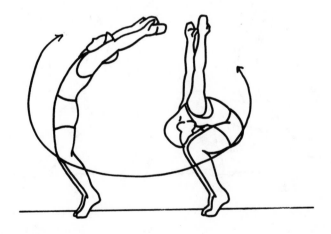

(b)

(c) *Split lunge waves.* Step forward with the right leg and bend it as much as possible while keeping the right foot on the floor and the left leg straight with the left foot on the floor. Sit back on the left leg, straighten right leg—10 repetitions, right and left.

(d) *Split lunge swings.* Step forward to a split lunge and then stand on the front leg and swing the back leg up. Swing back to original lunge position and repeat—10 repetitions, right and left.

(e) *Straddle lunge swings.* Step to a straddle lunge right and swing arms to right in a cross-and-swing pattern. Swing arms to left and follow with body to a straddle lunge left—10 repetitions.

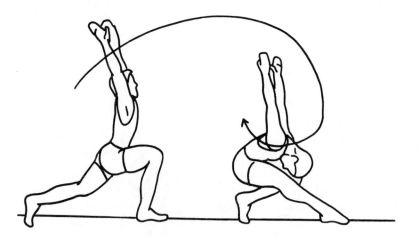

(c)

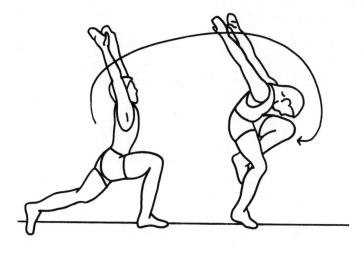

(d)

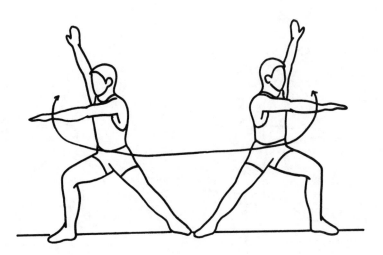

(e)

Rhythmic Leg Swings

(a) *Vertical forward and backward leg swing.* 10 repetitions, right and left.

(b) *Horizontal forward and backward leg swing.* 10 repetitions, right and left.

(c) *Forward leg circles.* 10 repetitions, right and left.

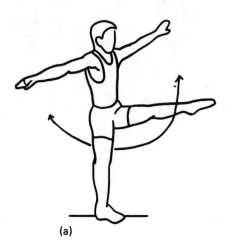

(a)

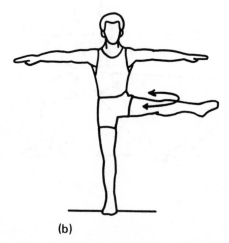

(b)

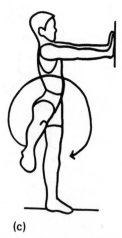

(c)

(d) Backward leg circles. 10 repetitions, right and left.
(e) Lateral leg swings. 10 repetitions, right and left.
(f) Knee scale vertical swings. 10 repetitions, right and left.
(g) Knee scale lateral swings. 10 repetitions, right and left.
(h) Knee scale leg circles. 10 repetitions, forward and back-ward, right and left.

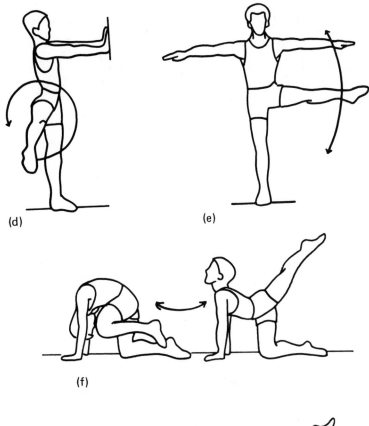

(d)

(e)

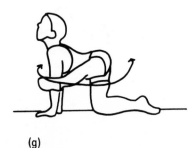

(f)

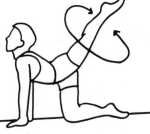

(g)

(h)

(i) Arch rise combination. 10 repetitions.

(j) Ankles. Sit and rotate the ankles 10 times each direction. Use hands to apply some force if desired.

(k) Seated, straddle arch swings. 5 repetitions, right and left.

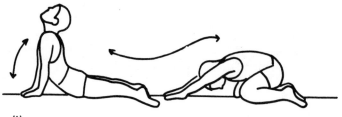

(i)

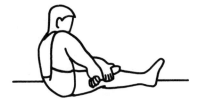

(j)

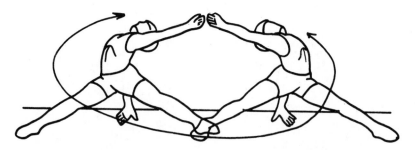

(k)

Static Flexibility Exercises

Stimulate Circulation

Begin the program with one to five minutes of brisk walking, jogging, cycling, or rope skipping to increase the heart rate to over 100 beats per minute.

Finger and Wrist Exercises

(a) Interlock the fingers, turn the palms away from the body, straighten the arms, and stretch for 3 seconds.

(b) Press the palms together and stretch the wrists. Hold for 3 seconds.

(c) Press the backs of the hands together and stretch the wrists. Hold for 3 seconds.

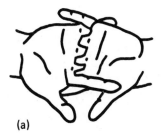

(a)

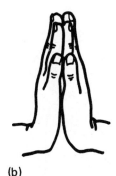

(b)

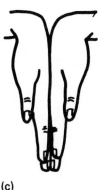

(c)

Elbow Flex

Extend and flex each elbow. Hold each position for 3 seconds.

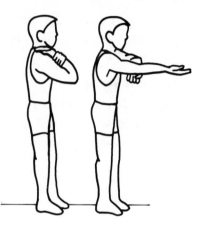

Shoulders

(a) Cross arms in front of body and grasp opposite shoulders. Create stretch tension and hold 3 seconds.

(b) Place right elbow behind head and use left hand to create stretch tension. Hold 3 seconds. Repeat with left elbow.

(c) Place one hand over head and behind back. Place the other hand in small of back. Try to join hands, create stretch tension and hold 3 seconds. Repeat to other side.

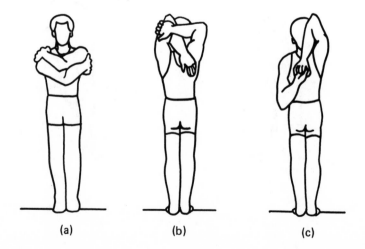

(a)   (b)   (c)

Neck

  (a) Lay head on left shoulder—hold 3 seconds.

  (b) Lay head on right shoulder—hold 3 seconds.

  (c) Turn chin to left shoulder—hold 3 seconds.

  (d) Turn chin to right shoulder—hold 3 seconds.

  (e) Pull head as far forward as possible and put chin on chest —hold 3 seconds.

  (f) Pull head back as far as possible, touching the back of the head to the shoulders—hold 3 seconds.

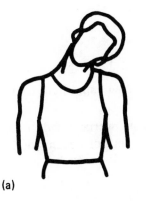

(a)

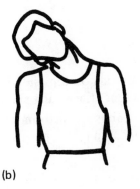

(b)

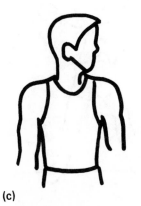

(c)

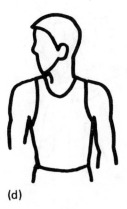

(d)

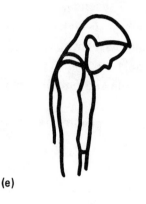

(e)

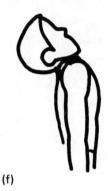

(f)

Trunk

(a) Hands on hips-side bends—3 seconds and hold each side 3 to 5 repetitions each side.

(b) Hands clasped and straight arms overhead-side bends—3 seconds and hold each side 3 to 5 repetitions each side.

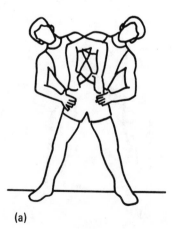

(a)

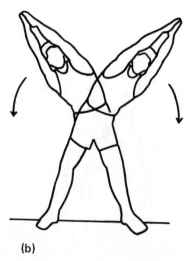

(b)

Legs/Back: Straddle Standing

  (a) Reach down the right—hold 3 seconds.

  (b) Reach down the left—hold 3 seconds.

  (c) Reach down the middle—hold 3 seconds.

  (d) Repeat each 3 times.

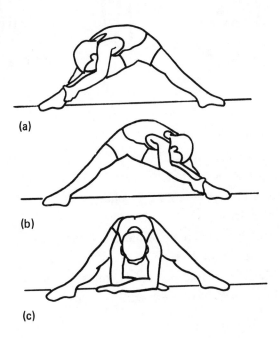

(a)

(b)

(c)

Legs/Back: Straight Standing

  (a) Squat stand—hold 1 second.

  (b) Stoop stand—hold 3 seconds.

  (c) Repeat each 3 times.

  (d) Pike stand—hold 3 seconds.

  (e) Repeat pike stand 3 times.

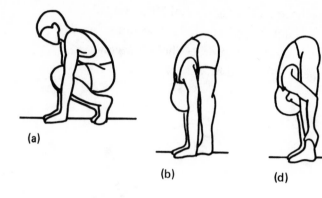

(a)

(b)

(d)

Back: All Fours/On Front

(a) Arch the back—hold 3 seconds.
(b) Round the back—hold 3 seconds.
(c) Knee scale right—hold 3 seconds.
(d) Knee scale left—hold 3 seconds.
(e) Knee and forehead sit—hold 3 seconds.
(f) Arch rise—hold 3 seconds.
(g) On the front—hold 3 seconds, relax.
(h) Arch rise, bent knees—hold 3 seconds.

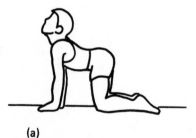

(a)

(b)

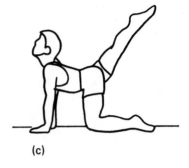

(c)

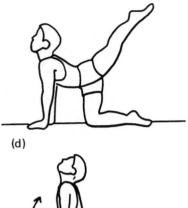

(d)

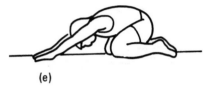

(e)

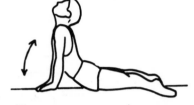
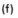

(f)

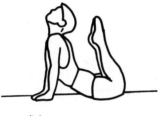

(h)

Back: On Front

(a) Right leg rise—hold 3 seconds.

(b) Left leg rise—hold 3 seconds.

(c) Right leg rise, cross and touch left hand—hold 3 seconds.

(d) Left leg rise, cross and touch right hand—hold 3 seconds.

(e) Full body arch—hold 3 seconds.

(f) Straddle full body arch—hold 3 seconds.

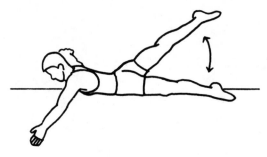

(a)

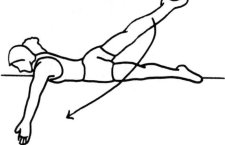

(b)

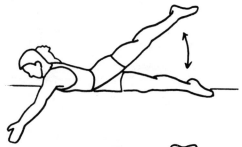

(c)

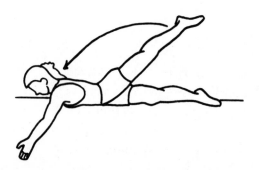

(d)

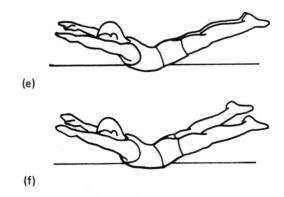

(e)

(f)

Ankles, Legs, Back: Straight Sit

(a) Flex right ankle, use hands to apply stretch tension—hold 3 seconds.

(b) Extend right ankle—hold 3 seconds.

(c) Flex left ankle—hold 3 seconds.

(d) Extend left ankle—hold 3 seconds.

(e) Single leg tuck sit right—hold 3 seconds.

(f) Single leg tuck straddle right using hands to pull knee to chest—hold 3 seconds.

(g) Single leg tuck straddle sit, right, leg on floor, reach down left leg and hold—3 seconds.

(h) Repeat (e), (f), and (g) on left.

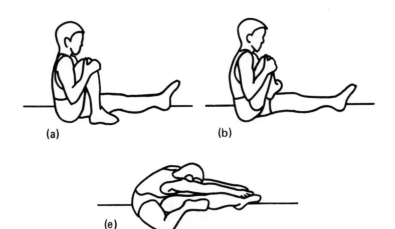

(a)   (b)

(e)

(i) Tuck straddle sit, hold hands on feet, pull down middle and hold—3 seconds.

(j) Pike sit—3 seconds.

(k) Pike sit, flexed ankle—3 seconds.

(l) Single leg, lift right—3 seconds.

(m) Single leg, lift left—3 seconds.

(n) Repeat (l) and (m) with ankles flexed.

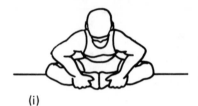

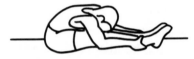

(i)

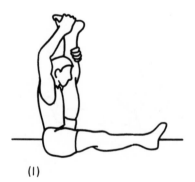

(j)

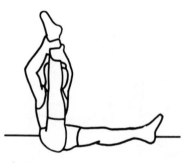

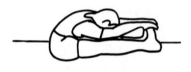

(k)

(l)

(m)

Legs/Back: On Back

    (a) Split lying right—3 seconds.

    (b) Split lying left—3 seconds.

    (c) Half pike lying right, cross right leg to left hand—3 seconds.

    (d) Half pike lying left, cross left leg to right hand—3 seconds.

    (e) Half pike lying, cross both legs to left, then right—3 seconds.

    (f) Deep tuck lying—3 seconds.

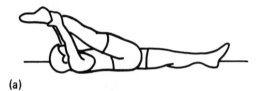

(a)

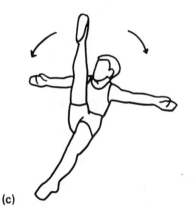

(c)

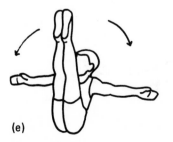

(e)

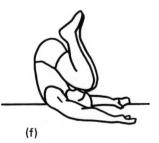

(f)

(g) Deep pike lying—3 seconds.

(h) Deep straddle, lying—3 seconds.

(i) Back arch stand—3 seconds (repeat with right leg, lift, then left—3 seconds each).

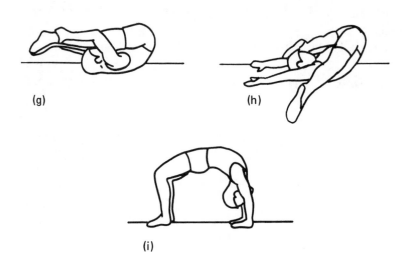

(g)   (h)

(i)

Legs/Back: Straddle Sit and Hurdler's Sit, Knee Stand

(a) *Straddle sit.* Reach right, left and middle—3 seconds each.

(b) *Hurdler's sit.* Reach right, middle, left, then lie back—3 seconds each. Repeat with left leg straight and right leg bent.

(c) *Knee stand.* Quad stretch lean—4 times increasing distance each time—3 seconds hold each.

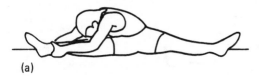

(a)

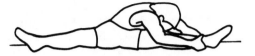

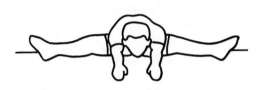

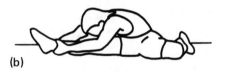

(b)

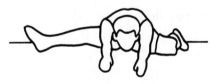

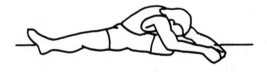

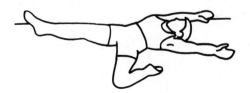

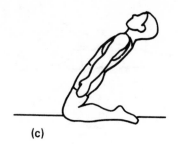

(c)

Legs/Straddle Stand

(a) Straddle lunge right — 3 seconds.
(b) Straddle lunge left—3 seconds.
(c) Wide squat straddle stand—3 seconds.
(d) Split lunge right—3 seconds.
(e) Split lunge left—3 seconds.
(f) Straight leg split lunge right—3 seconds.
(g) Straight leg split lunge left—3 seconds.

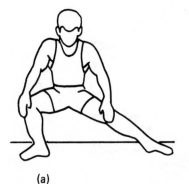
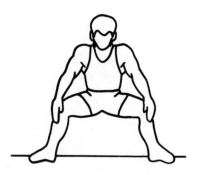

(a)   (c)

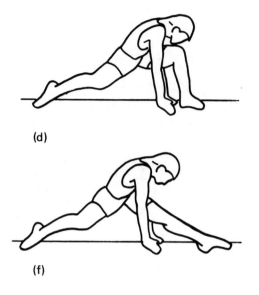

(d)

(f)

Splits

(a) Split right—3 seconds.
(b) Split left—3 seconds.
(c) Wide straddle sit—3 seconds.
(d) Wide straddle on front—3 seconds.
(e) Repeat (a), (b), (c), and (d).

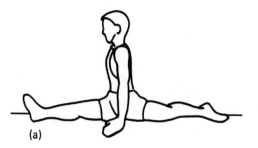

(a)

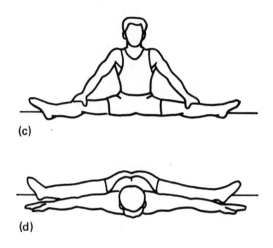

(c)

(d)

Shoulders/Sit

   (a) Reach back with left hand—3 seconds.
   (b) Reach back with right hand—3 seconds.
   (c) Reach back both hands—3 seconds.

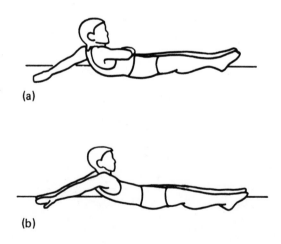

(a)

(b)

Calf/Achilles Tendon Stretch

Use slant board. Stand on slant board, hands against wall.
Hold for 3 seconds on right foot, 3 seconds on left. Repeat.

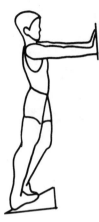

Resistive Flexibility Exercises

Back: Arch and Round

Partner puts resistance on mid-back of performer. Perform
10 arch and rounds.

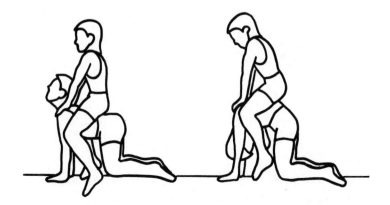

Anterior Leg and Hip Stretch

Performer lies on front. Five presses each leg. Start easy and low; progress to hard and high.

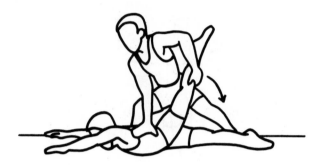

Quad Stretch

Performer lies on front. Five presses each leg. Start easy and progress to harder presses. Try to touch heel to rear before final press.

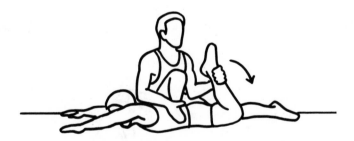

Hamstring Presses

(a) Performer lies on back. Five presses from 90-degree angle to floor each leg. Each press progressively harder.

(b) Five each leg. Press from positions greater than 90 degrees to 90-degree starting point. Start easy and progress to harder presses. Start with 100 degree and progress to maximum tolerance.

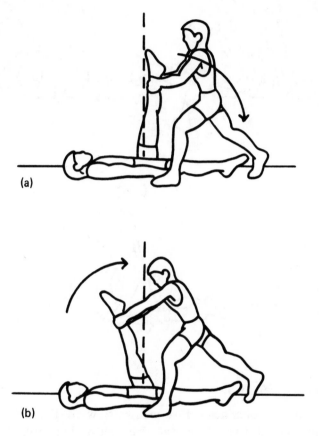

(a)

(b)

Abductor, Adductor Presses

(a) *Tuck sit.* Partner holds knees. Five presses outward, five inward.

(b) *Tuck lying.* Partner holds knees. Five presses outward, five inward.

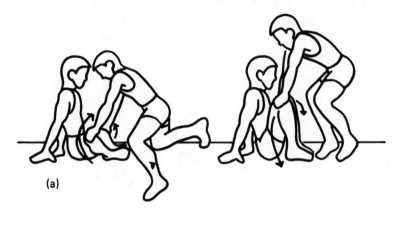

(a)

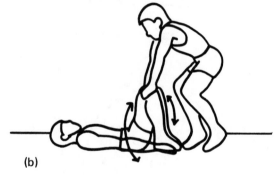

(b)

Neck: Straight Sit

Partner holds head. Five presses forward, five backward, five right lateral, five left lateral, five right-to-left turns, five left-to-right turns.

Shoulders/Arms: Straight Sit

(a) *Straight arm.* Partner holds arms. Five forward depressions, five forward elevations, five lateral depressions, five lateral elevations, five forward-and-horizontal presses, five rear-and-horizontal presses.

(b) *Bent arm.* Partner holds elbows. Hands behind head. Five forward horizontal presses, five rear horizontal presses.

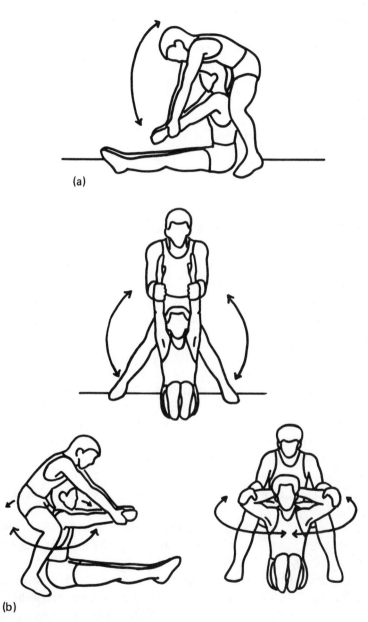

(a)

(b)

Foot Flexors and Extensors

Straight sit, partner holds feet. Five ankle extensions and five ankle flexions.

2

Strength Training

Generally speaking, *strength* is the ability of a muscle to exert tension against a resistance. Strength is usually measured by the amount of resistance a muscle can overcome. In specific relation to muscle responsiveness, *fundamental strength* is the ability of the muscle or muscle set to exert sufficient tension to move its related body part through the complete range of movement without assistance from an unrelated muscle or muscle set. *Refined strength* is the ability of the muscle or muscle set to move its related body part plus as much additional body weight resistance as possible through that same range of motion under the same circumstances.

The concept of muscle responsiveness also recognized a third type of strength—*specialized* or *limited-range strength*. Specialized strength is the ability of a muscle to overcome high levels of resistance, usually within a limited range of motion, yet still without assistance from an unrelated muscle or muscle set. Specialized strength is often the greatest problem area in strength development, for it often makes the rest of the muscle weak in relation to a specific area of the muscle. Although specialized strength is necessary in sport, muscle responsiveness is at its peak when the difference between specialized strength and refined strength is minimal. When an athlete seeks to develop specialized strength, he or she should use the training devices that develop as much of the whole range of movement as possible.

Strength in any range is dependent on the proper functioning of all motor unit elements. A motor unit is composed of a ventral horn cell, its motor nerve fiber, and those muscle fibers that it enervates. There are many motor units in a muscle and strength of a muscle is proportional to the number of motor units in action at a specific time and also the frequency of motor unit stimulation within the realm of training. Therefore, proper application of training principles can increase strength by increasing the involvement of motor units. Strength performance of a muscle is also directly related to the following:

Nutrition. A balanced diet which provides essential growth, maintenance, and repair needs constitutes good nutrition. The best advice any athlete can receive comes from his or her doctor and any nutritional expert recommended by the doctor. Do not follow fad diets prescribed by nonprofessionals.

Rest. The more intense the strength training, the greater the need for rest between exercise sessions. As a general rule, overload strength training should be scheduled every thirty-six to forty-eight hours. Consult your coach, trainer, and doctor for your specific needs.

Age and gender. Check with your trainer and doctor to be sure that your strength goals are reasonable for you. Strength for the young is a function of maturity. Young adults generally gain greater proportionate amounts of strength than the rest of the adult population; men generally gain greater proportionate amounts of strength than women. The potential for strength gain among women athletes is almost totally unknown. Women athletes may be able to equal and even surpass male athletes in strength someday. Women who seek to accomplish this goal safely should consult first with the best professional advice.

Psychological and emotional factors. Your personal state of psychological and emotional readiness during training may determine whether you maintain, increase, or decrease your strength. Try to concentrate and be consistent in your approach to strength training. Try not to let external or internal disturbances interfere with your strength workout.

Efficient removal of fatigue products. Always increase circulation before strength exercises and use exercises that promote good cardiovascular functioning. Excessive overloads and isometric exercises often disturb proper circulation and may even harm the cardiovascular system. Check with your doctor to be certain of the value of your strength exercise program.

Always precede your strength program with a good warmup emphasizing flexibility exercises, and intersperse flexibility exercises with your strength exercises. Finish your workout with a good warmdown maintaining a stepped-up circulation while effectively stretching the muscles you've used. Strength exercises tempered with flexibility exercises promote good cardiovascular functioning and improved circulation in the capillary networks. The body becomes more efficient in removing muscular fatigue products. This improves strength training effects, maintains flexibility, reduces soreness, and helps lower the injury potential.

Mechanical factors of leverage. Exercise the muscle or muscle sets in their natural patterns of movement. Let them operate their respective lever systems properly. Placing a muscle or muscle set in a position of mechanical disadvantage simply causes strain and may promote injury.

There are thousands of methods for developing strength. They range from free calisthenics to the use of an ever-increasing number of sophisticated machines. Each method seems to have its own theory and its own school of physiologists who guarantee the success of that particular method. Amid all the conflicting evidence and claims, everyone accepts some fundamentals. One of these fundamentals is that there are two ways a muscle contracts—isometrically and isotonically. Isometric contraction means that a muscle exerts tension against a resistance without changing the positioned length of a muscle. Proponents of isometrics say that these exercises produce great strength gains in specific areas of the muscles and, when applied to critical positions throughout the full range of motion, produce high-level strength in the entire muscle. Detractors of isometrics question the quality of the strength gain and claim stress on the heart and blood pressure.

Isotonic contraction is more complex. Basically it means that a muscle shortens (concentric contraction) or lengthens (eccentric contraction) when exerting tension against a resistance. Resistance may be in the form of a *fixed workload*, one which remains the same through the entire exercise, or an *accommodating workload*, one which changes to meet the appropriate needs of each muscle length during the entire exercise. Because isotonic exercise is the most common method of strength exercise, proponents and detractors abound. Research evidence, pro and con, may be found virtually anywhere one finds an article about strength exercise.

Isotonic exercises applied to the full range of motion (as developed by flexibility exercises) is the method of strength gain advocated by this text. The programs for strength development for muscle responsiveness use mostly the weight of the body part, the weight of body areas, and sometimes the weight of the whole body. An elemental program for specialized strength is also included. Beyond these the athlete must seek out advanced modern weight training devices to meet his needs.

Here are some of the methods of isotonic strength exercises with a guiding comment about each:

Concentric contraction using body weight to develop fundamental and refined strength. The idea here is to use basic full-range movement patterns with resistance coming only from gravity and the weight of the related body part. The method of overload is that of traditional calisthenics and modern gymnastics: increase the gravitational disadvantage and the amount of body weight to increase the resistance for each movement. Development of fundamental strength by moving the related body part through its entire range gradually changes to development of refined strength. Refined strength is controlling as much of the entire body weight as possible within sound mechanical and anatomical limits. The variables involved in these two approaches permit natural occurrences of both fixed and accommodating workloads. The objective is to produce full range movement that effectively controls one's own body weight before trying to control resistance greater than body weight.

Concentric contraction with a fixed workload for specialized strength. This method utilizes primarily free weights and possibly some form of modern weight training machines of the athlete's choice. It produces high-level strength gains but demands a disciplined program with a variety of exercises if the athlete wishes to keep strength reasonably balanced through the entire range of movement.

Concentric contraction with accommodating workload for specialized strength. This method utilizes modern exercise machines which have levers, pulleys, gears, chains, and even hydraulics to adjust the workload to the needs of the muscle during various phases of the exercise. It produces high-level strength gains through most of the entire range but demands intense training to keep that balance while also developing the specialized strength the athlete seeks. Its greatest disadvantage is that it requires expensive and exclusive machinery, which is all too often unavailable to the athlete.

Eccentric contraction with a fixed workload for specialized strength. This method utilizes free weights and some forms of machines. Because it requires lengthening of the muscle against a resistance, it also requires a partner for assistance and safety. It does produce extremely high levels of specialized strength in a short time, but it is dangerous to the muscles, the skeletal structure, and the cardiovascular system. It also may not be effective through the entire range.

Eccentric contraction with accommodating workload for specialized strength. This method utilizes the most exclusive modern exercise machines and often requires a partner for assistance. Safety features are generally built into the machine. This method produces extremely high levels of specialized strength in a short time, but it may also be dangerous to the muscles, the skeletal structure, and the cardiovascular system. It has the additional disadvantage of requiring expensive exclusive machinery.

Here are several programs of strength exercises that will help the athlete attain sufficient strength gains to easily handle his body weight. They are in keeping with the concept of muscle responsiveness. If the athlete wishes to build specialized strength beyond these levels, he or she must seek the guidance of weight training experts. *However, even in weight training, the concepts and guidelines that rule muscle responsiveness still apply.*

Concentric Contraction Exercises

Review the static flexibility exercises in chapter 2. Try to perform one of each exercise through the entire range *free*—that is, no aid from other body parts, no hands to help leg lifts, etc. When you can do all exercises correctly and freely, you have reached the level of *fundamental strength*. The first level of *refined strength* comes when you can do the following program. The next step is to use the principles of training to increase the intensity of the refined strength program.

A third option that enhances both fundamental and refined strength development is to get a partner and perform the resistive flexibility workout with as much resistance as you can effectively handle.

1. Precede this program with an effective warmup emphasizing increased circulation and flexibility exercises.

2. Begin the program with exercises for the back, legs, and shoulders.

(a) Lie on your front and perform the following:

(1) 5 free arch rises.

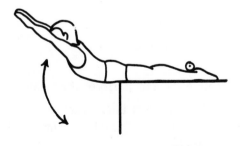

(I)

(2) 5 lower body rises.

(3) 5 full body arches.

(4) 5 straddle full body arches.

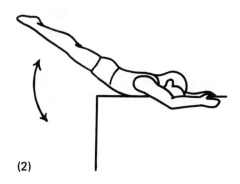

(2)

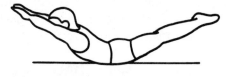

(3)

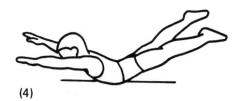

(4)

(b) Lie on your back and perform the following:

(1) 5 shoulder support back arches.

(2) 5 head support back arches, arms on floor.

(3) 5 back arches.

(4) 4 single leg back arches, 2 right and 2 left.

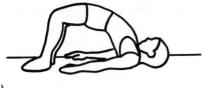

(1)

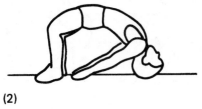

(2)

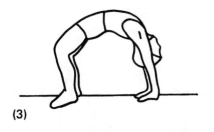

(3)

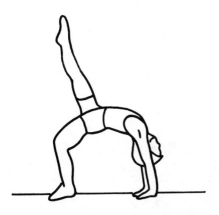

(4)

(5) 5 overgrip dislocate to arch stands using a wand.

(6) 5 undergrip dislocate to arch stands using a wand.

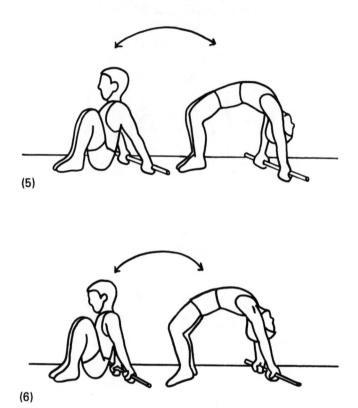

(5)

(6)

3. Abdominal and Hip Flexor Exercises

(a) 5 touch sit-ups.

(b) 6 alternate elbow touch sit-ups.

(c) 5 V sit-ups.

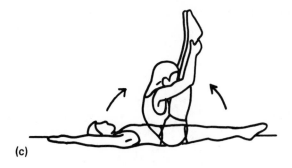

(c)

4. 10 Lateral Double Leg Crossovers while Lying on Back
5. 5 Deep Pike Leg Lifts
6. 5 Deep Straddle Leg Lifts

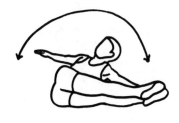

(4)

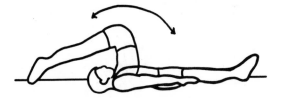

(5)

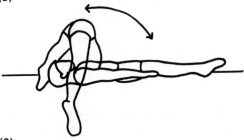

(6)

7. 5 Seated Single Leg Lifts, 3 per leg—hold 1 second
8. 5 Straddle Leg Slides
9. 5 Half Pike Lying Leg Straddles—hold 1 second

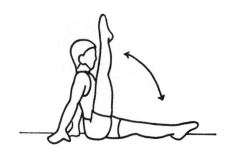

(7)

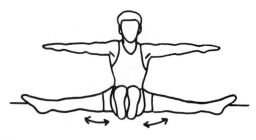

(8)

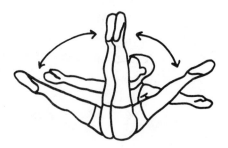

(9)

10. 5 Split Lying Single Leg Lifts, 3 each leg—hold 1 second

11. 5 Tuck Sit Leg Straddles

12. 5 Free Pike Sits

13. 5 Free Straddle Pike Sits

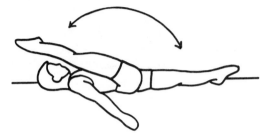

(10)

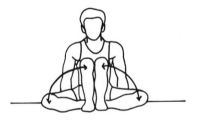

(11)

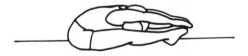

(12)

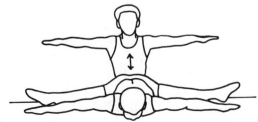

(13)

14. 5 Quad Leans from Knee Stand—hold 1 second

15. 6 Side Arches—3 each side

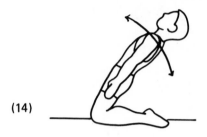

(14)

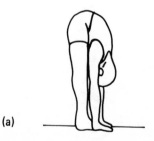

(15)

16. Standing:

(a) 5 free pike stands. Hold head to knees 1 second.

(b) 9 free pike straddle stands—right, left, middle—3 each.

(c) 5 squats.

(d) 3 single leg squats, right and left.

(e) 3 free leg curls each leg, lean against wall, touch heel to rear and hold 1 second.

(a)

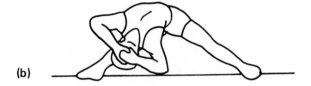

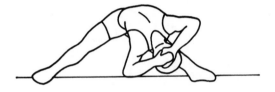

(b)

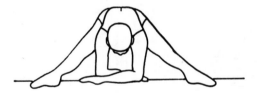

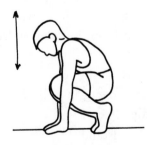

(c)

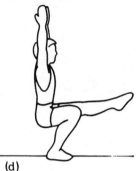

(d)

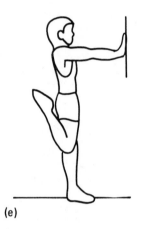

(e)

17. Arms, Shoulders, Chest

(a) 5 push-ups, floor.

(b) 5 parallel bar or chair dip push-ups.

(c) 1 straddle leg, 1 arm push-up each arm.

(d) 1 straight arm push-up, arms extended overhead.

(e) 5 overgrip pull-ups.

(f) 5 undergrip chins.

(g) 5 behind the neck overgrip pull-ups.

(h) 5 handstand dips-floor.

(i) 5 parallel bar handstand dips.

(j) 5 L hangs or leg raises while hanging.

(k) 1 overgrip skin the cat hang and pull backout.

(l)　1 undergrip skin the cat hang and pull backout.

(m) 5 parallel bar dips.

(n)　1 20-foot rope climb using arms only.

18. Partner assisted neck and shoulder exercises and ankle flex-extended exercises—as listed in resistive flexibility program but with more resistance: 5 each.

19. Complete the program with a good warmdown emphasizing circulation increase and flexibility exercises.

3

Speed Training

Contrary to popular belief, speed is not simply a natural attribute. Certainly, speed is limited by your genetic capacity for neuromuscular action, as well as body structure, but athletes seldom reach their potential for speed and its related response, quickness. Speed and quickness are really skills—the skills of rapid force application to the body's leverage system.

Because of the multiple leverage systems formed by the skeleton and skeletal muscles, and also the predominance of first- and third-class levers with their short-power arms, the human body is designed for speed and quickness rather than overcoming resistance. Therefore, an individual's potential for speed and quickness can be developed by improving his skill in four areas of force application: (1) amount of force applied, (2) direction in which the force is applied, (3) the point at which the force is applied, and (4) the duration of the force application. An individual's potential for speed and quickness can only be reached by developing strength through the full range of motion and then using proper force application to master specific skills. An untrained and unskilled individual may run a race or perform a quickness test many times at random and never reveal his true potential for speed or quickness. The same may often be true for a conditioned athlete performing the skills of his sport if he has not mastered the intricate force application techniques that comprise the sport skills.

The concept of muscle responsiveness holds that the best way to start to develop speed and quickness is to apply strength to the full range of motion. The exercises in chapters 2 and 3 become very important to the individual seeking to improve speed and quickness. The next step is to learn to perform those exercises quickly, first performing only one repetition and then performing as many repetitions as possible in a short period of time. The basic idea is to learn to control the body weight, whether it is the weight of a specific body part or the weight of the entire body. For some exercises the athlete may choose to add small amounts of additional weight to overload the muscle. The athlete must practice natural movement patterns, progressively increasing the number of correct performances he can do in short periods of time. Thus, speed and quickness exercises become a natural outgrowth of flexibility and strength training.

Speed and quickness for any athletic skill can be developed by breaking down the skill into its fundamental movement patterns and working on these patterns with flexibility, strength, and speed exercises. Athletes generally learn a skill in its gross forms and only break it down when there is a coordination problem. *Muscle responsiveness comes when the parts of a skill become fundamental movement patterns used in conditioning exercises, including speed exercises.* This approach may help the athlete learn his skill better by giving him an improved insight into the nature of the skill. However, the primary objective is to improve the responsiveness of the muscles involved in the necessary specific movement patterns.

Breaking down a skill into fundamental movement patterns begins with biomechanical skill analysis through the disciplines of kinematics and kinetics.

Kinematics is the analysis of the individual's physical structure and his personal biomechanical approach to a skill problem. Kinematic analysis reveals the geometry of the individual's leverage system including the length of power and weight arms, the position of the fulcrum, the most efficient method of force application, the necessary amount and duration of force application, and the point of force application needed for the levers involved in the specific skill. Kinematic analysis reveals the specific flexibility, strength, and force application techniques you must work on to improve your speed and quickness performances for specific skills.

Kinetics is the analysis of the specific skill and it deals with force, mass, energy, and their effect on motion. Kinetics helps the individual understand the skill he wishes to perform. Understanding kinetics begins with Newton's laws of inertia, acceleration, and reaction.

The comments on biomechanical analysis have been included here because speed and quickness are two predominant characteristics of quality athletic performance. They often are the sole indicators of an athlete's capabilities to coaches. Many great athletes have failed in the sports world simply because they didn't understand how to reach their potential for speed and quickness. To do so you must understand your skill areas, how your body can best produce these specific skills, and how to break these skills down into basic movement patterns for conditioning exercises. By increasing muscle responsiveness with skill-related speed exercises, the athlete can improve his training and practice techniques and reach his potential for speed and quickness for specific skills.

Coaches, trainers, doctors, and researchers knowledgeable in biomechanics are helping more and more athletes perform faster and quicker. These same athletes would once have been passed over because they didn't appear fast or quick at first testing or because they didn't improve training methods as they got older. In many sports, an athlete may perform well into his forties without much loss of speed or quickness if he maintains proper conditioning.

Big-Muscle Program for Building Speed and Quickness

Stimulate Circulation

Begin the program with an effective warmup that steps up circulation and emphasizes flexibility exercises.

Exercises from Hands-and-Knees Position

(a) *Arch and round.* One time as fast as possible, then as many times as possible in 5 seconds.

(b) *Knee scale swings.* One time right and left, then for 5 seconds, each side.

(c) *Side knee scale swings.* One time right and left, then 5 seconds, each side.

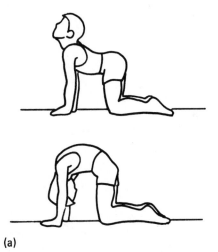

(a)

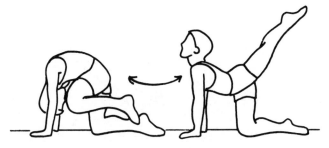

(b)

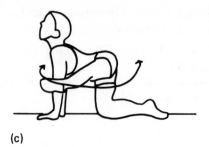

(c)

Exercises in the Prone Position

(a) *Arch rise combination.* One time, then for 5 seconds.

(b) *Single leg rise and crossover.*

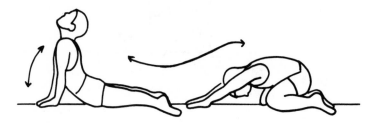

(a)

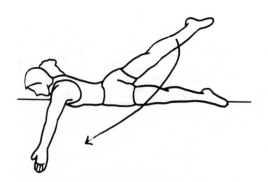

(b)

(c) *Full body arch.*

(d) *Straddle full body arch.*

(e) *Bird's nest or cradle arch.*

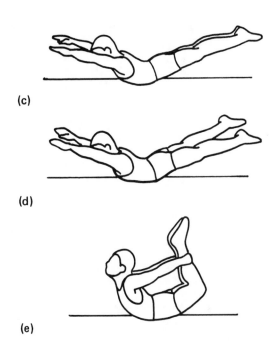

(c)

(d)

(e)

Exercises in the Back Arch Stand Position

(a) From hook lying, explode to back arch stand. One time as fast as possible, then as many times as possible within 5 seconds.

(b) From hook lying, explode to single leg back arch stand. One time as fast as possible, right, then left. Then right as many times as possible within 5 seconds, then left for 5 seconds.

(c) From single leg back arch stand, perform single leg swings. One time as fast as possible, right, then left. Then right as many times as possible within 5 seconds, then left for 5 seconds.

Note: These exercises may be modified if necessary by using either the shoulder support arch stand or the head and arms support arch stand.

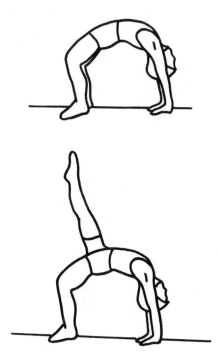

Exercises in the Seated Position

(a) *Straddle swing slides.* One time, then for 5 seconds.

(b) *Tuck straddle swings.* One time, then for 5 seconds.

(c) *Straddle arch right and left.* One time, then for 5 seconds.

(d) *Right, left, and middle from straddle sit.* One time, then for 10 seconds.

(e) *Pike sit.* One time, then for 5 seconds.

(f) *Double leg tuck sit swings.* One time, then for 10 seconds.

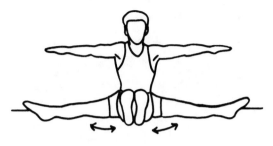

(a)

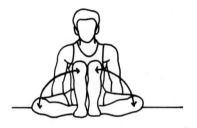

(b)

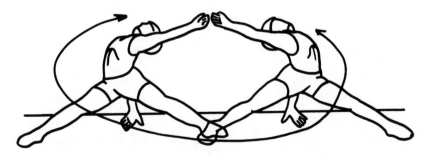

(c)

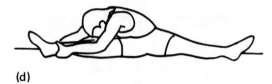

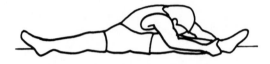

(d)

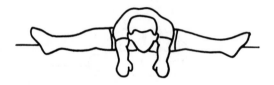

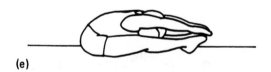

(e)

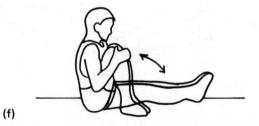

(f)

Exercises on the Back

(a) *Double leg tuck lying swings.* One time, then for 10 seconds.

(b) *Single leg lifts.* One time, right and left, then for 5 seconds right and for 5 seconds left.

(c) *Double leg lifts to deep pike.* One time, then for 5 seconds.

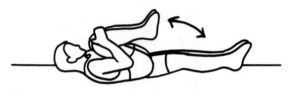

(a)

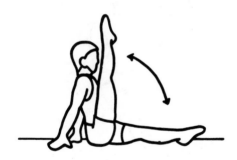

(b)

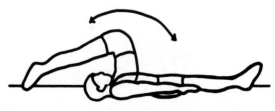

(c)

(d) *Double leg lifts to deep straddle.* One time, then for 5 seconds.

(e) *Single leg crossovers.* One time, right and left—each leg. Then for 5 seconds each leg.

(f) *Double leg crossovers.* One time, then for 5 seconds.

(g) *Double leg tuck crossovers.* One time, then for 5 seconds.

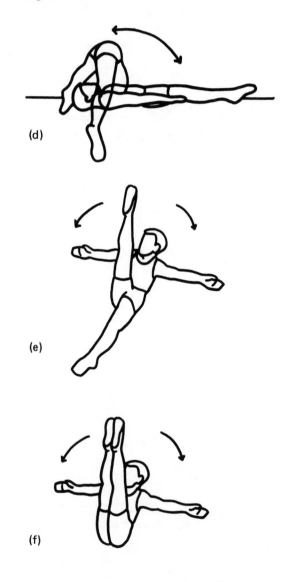

(d)

(e)

(f)

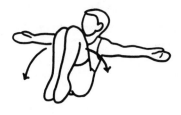

(g)

Arm Exercises

Lie on back and hold a two- to five-pound weight in each hand.

(a) *Crossovers*. One time, then for 5 seconds.

(b) *Bent arm shoulder rotations*. One time, then for 5 seconds.

(c) *Lateral arm slides*. One time, then for 5 seconds.

(d) *Frontal arm swings*. One time, then for 5 seconds.

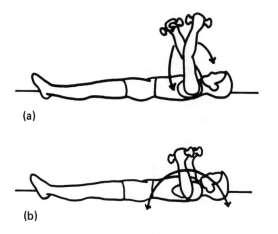

(a)

(b)

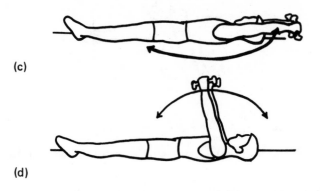

(c)

(d)

Abdominal and Hip Flexor Exercise while Lying on Back

(a) *Free tuck sit-up.* One time, then for 5 seconds.
(b) *Free V sit-up.* One time, then for 5 seconds.
(c) *Free straddle V sit-up.* One time, then for 5 seconds.

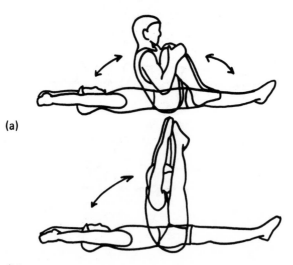

(a)

(b)

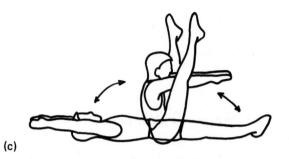

(c)

Arms, Shoulders, and Chest Exercises

One time, then for 5 seconds:
- (a) *Simple push-up.*
- (b) *Parallel bar dip.*
- (c) *Handstand push-up.*
- (d) *Parallel bar push-up—deep.*
- (e) *Undergrip chin.*
- (f) *Overgrip pull-up.*
- (g) *Overgrip pull-up behind neck.*
- (h) *10-foot rope climb for speed.* Free, no legs, from sit.

Abdominal and Hip Flexor Exercises from Hang

(a) *Single leg lifts.* One time each, right and left. Then each for 5 seconds.

(b) *Double leg lifts.* One time, then for 5 seconds.

(c) *Double leg lifts straddled.* One time, then for 5 seconds.

Neck Exercises

A simple and safe way to apply speed exercises to the neck is to go to the shallow area of a swimming pool, stand on the bottom, submerge the head and perform lateral, forward-backward, and turning movements using the water as both resistance and cushion.

Weight Exercises

Any exercise performed with free weights or on an exercise machine can become a speed exercise simply by cutting the resistance to a very small amount, for instance, only the weight of the bar.

Warmdown

Conclude this program with a thorough warmdown emphasizing circulation and flexibility exercises.

Warning: Do not try this program until you have prepared your muscles with several weeks of flexibility and strength training. *Also, the exercises here, if improperly performed, can turn out to be nothing more than bouncing flexibility exercises. Keep all movements in control. Do not bounce them.* Move through each exercise in a fluid manner, *paying attention to good form.*

4

Endurance Training

Endurance is defined as performance ability for extended periods of time. Endurance may be more broadly defined as stress tolerance and broken down into four basic categories:

1. *Basic or daily living endurance.* The ability to expend a continual but low level of energy sufficient to maintain normal body functions and muscular well-being at rest and to tolerate the simple physical stress of daily life.

2. *Moderate or steady state endurance.* The ability to pace an expenditure of energy sufficient to tolerate a constant physical stress at a constant rate for a prolonged period of time.

3. *Maximum or exhaustive endurance.* The ability to continue expending energy sufficient to tolerate an increasing physical stress that pushes physiological limits or results in complete exhaustion.

4. *Psychological endurance.* The ability to expend nervous energy sufficient to tolerate a physical stress plus the mental and emotional stress which accompany it.

Within this broader concept of endurance lies the concept of muscular endurance, the last component of muscle responsiveness. Muscular endurance is the ability of a muscle to sustain or repeat a contraction for a given length of time or until exhaustion. Muscular endurance cannot be separated from the larger concept of endurance. Muscular endurance is subordinate to organic stress tolerance—the functioning of the heart, lungs, vascular system, the kidneys, and all other organs. It is also subordinate to the stress tolerance of physique or body structure and mental and emotional stress tolerance, as well as the motivation-influenced behavior-regulating devices of will power, self-control, inhibition, initiative, and concentration. No area of muscle responsiveness demands more attention to the principles of training than muscular endurance, both physically and psychologically.

DEVELOPING MUSCULAR ENDURANCE

The development of muscular endurance encompasses most directly the principles of overload with special emphasis on repetition. The level of endurance attained is directly related to the intensity and duration of the repetitions. Both steady-state and exhaustive muscular endurance performed through the whole range of motion will produce a high level of muscle responsiveness and total endurance. They should prepare you for the greater endurance demands of your specific skills. In the process, they should also help prepare you to meet the endurance demands of your sport, although additional endurance work related to the whole game or activity is necessary.

The program of muscular endurance exercises presented here will serve as a complete training program for the novice but may be only a test that reveals fundamental weaknesses for the advanced athlete. In any case, this program is just a beginning. Each athlete will eventually have to apply the rules of training in more advanced ways to further increase his endurance level.

GUIDELINES FOR THE ENDURANCE PROGRAM

1. Prepare for this program for several weeks or more, using flexibility, strength, and speed exercises only.

2. Select only a few items from the program at first. Change items each day. Finally, add all exercises to the daily workload.

3. Always use a good warmup and warmdown to accompany the program.

4. Review the principles of training and use them to adjust and adapt the program to your needs and goals.

5. The prescribed times and repetitions are goals. Do not start with them, but rather progress toward them.

6. Exercises can be performed to exhaustion if you choose. The working definition of exhaustion is the inability to perform the exercise correctly.

Endurance Exercise Program

Warmup

Begin the program with a thorough warmup emphasizing increased circulation and flexibility exercises.

Exercises Using the Back Arch Stand

(a) *Back push-ups.* Perform for 30 seconds.

(b) *Rock back and forward in back arch stand.* Perform for 30 seconds.

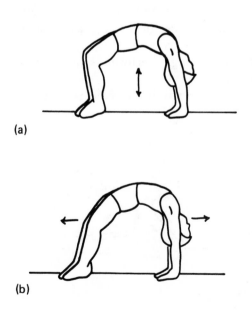

(a)

(b)

(c) *Single leg lifts from back arch stand.* Perform alternate right and left leg lifts for 30 seconds.

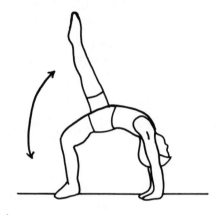

(c)

Exercises from Straight Sit

(a) *Tuck sits.* Perform as fast as possible for 30 seconds.

(b) *Tuck straddle sits.* Perform as fast as possible for 30 seconds.

(c) *Straddle slide swings.* Perform as fast as possible for 30 seconds.

(d) *Single leg lifts.* Perform alternate right and left leg lifts for 30 seconds.

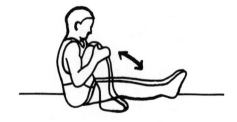

(a)

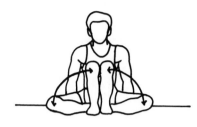

(b)

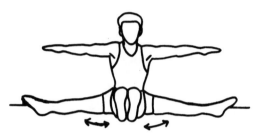

(c)

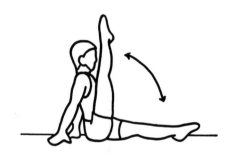

(d)

(e) *Leg circles.* Perform for 15 seconds in one direction and 15 seconds in other direction.

(f) *Single knee bends from straddle sit.* Perform alternate right and left knee bends for 30 seconds.

(g) *Reach right, left, middle from straddle sit.* Perform for 30 seconds each.

(h) *Pike Sits.* Perform for 30 seconds.

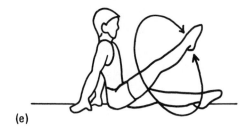

(e)

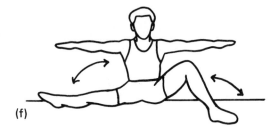

(f)

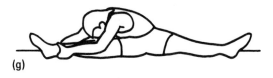

(g)

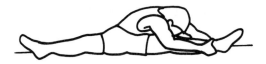

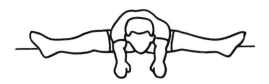

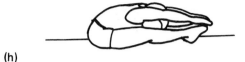

(h)

Exercises from Straight Lying

(a) *Single knee lifts.* Perform alternate right and left knee lifts for 30 seconds.

(b) *Double knee lifts to tuck lying.* Perform for 30 seconds.

(c) *Single leg lifts.* Perform alternate right and left leg lifts for 30 seconds.

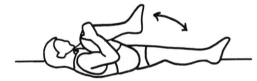

(a)

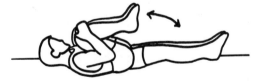

(b)

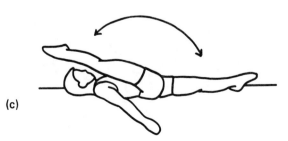

(c)

(d) *Double leg lifts to pike lying.* Perform for 30 seconds.

(e) *Double leg lifts to pike-straddle lying.* Perform for 30 seconds.

(f) *Lateral leg lifts to half-pike lying.* Perform for 30 seconds.

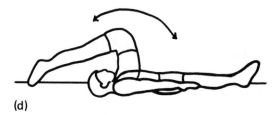

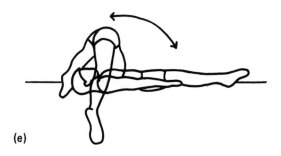

(d)

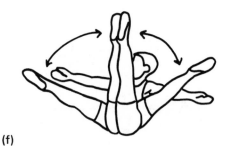

(e)

(f)

(g) *Leg circles.* Perform 15 seconds in one direction and 15 seconds in other direction.

(h) *Half-pike crossovers.* Perform for 30 seconds.

(i) *Hip circles.* Perform for 15 seconds in one direction then 15 seconds in other direction. Circle legs past arm, over head to deep pike, past other arm, to straight lying, and repeat.

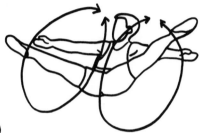

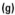

(g)

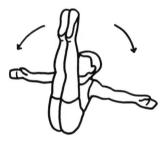

(h)

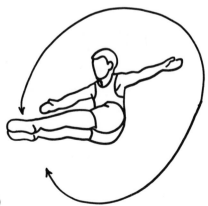

(i)

Exercises from On-Front

(a) *Arch rise combination.* Perform for 30 seconds.

(b) *Cradles.* Perform for 30 seconds.

(c) *Full body arches, closed and straddled.* Perform each for 15 seconds.

(d) *Single leg crossovers.* Perform 15 seconds right leg and 15 seconds left leg.

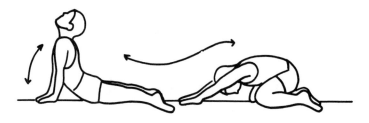

(a)

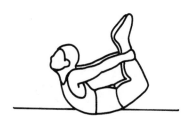

(b)

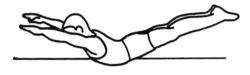

(c)

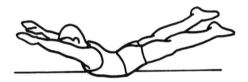

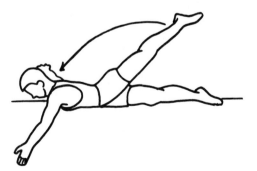

(d)

Exercises from Standing

(a) *Reach right, left, and middle.* Perform for 30 seconds.

(b) *Pike stands.* Perform for 30 seconds.

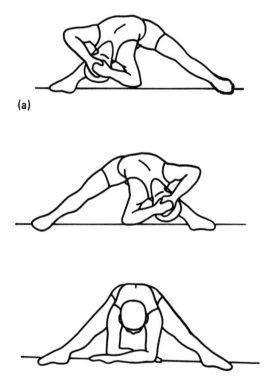

(a)

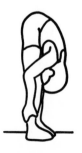

(b)

Additional Exercises

  (a) *Push-ups*—50 repetitions.
  (b) *Tuck sit-ups*—50 repetitions.
  (c) *V sit-ups*—50 repetitions.
  (d) *Straddle V sit-ups*—25 repetitions.
  (e) *P-bar dips*—30 repetitions.
  (f) *Overgrip pull-ups*—30 repetitions.
  (g) *Undergrip pull-ups*—30 repetitions.
  (h) *Squat jumps*—40 repetitions.
  (i) *Handstand presses*—15 repetitions.
  (j) *Back arch push-ups*—15 repetitions.
  (k) *From hanging, double leg lifts*—25 repetitions.
  (l) *From hanging, straddle double leg lifts*—25 repetitions.
  (m) *12-minute run, aiming for 2 miles.*
  (n) *Quad stretches*—20 repetitions.
  (o) *Single leg squats*—10 each leg.

Warmdown

Complete the program with an extensive warmdown, emphasizing flexibility exercises.

Warning: Do not try this program until you have prepared your muscles with several weeks of flexibility and strength training. *Also, the exercises here, if improperly performed, can turn out to be nothing more than bouncing flexibility exercises. Keep all movements in control. Do not bounce them.* Move through each exercise in a fluid manner, *paying attention to good form.*

Part Two

Refining Muscle Responsiveness

5

Basic Movement Patterns

Performance of all the exercises in Part One develops muscle responsiveness but leaves the individual only a crude athlete. He must now embark on a long journey through basic movement patterns that will refine his muscle power, hone, and polish it, and mold him into a capable athlete ready for the specific skills of his chosen athletic career.

In this section many of the most important basic movement patterns are presented. Mastery of these patterns will give an individual new insights relating to his athletic prowess. They will also suggest other areas he may wish or need to explore and also master if he wants to be a total athlete. The roots of athletic skills can be found in gymnastics, the foundation of all sports. The complete athletic development attained from tumbling, trampoline, and gymnastic apparatus work is of immeasurable importance to all athletes.

FUNDAMENTAL SKILLS

Running Skills

1. *Form Running*

(a) Forward with long even strides—various distances

(b) Forward with short powerful strides—various distances up to 220 yards

    (c) Backward running—various short distances

    (d) Slide step lateral running—various short distances

    (e) Carioca lateral running—various short distances

    (f) Running while twisting—various short distances

2. *Speed Running*

    (a) Forward—record speed for 10, 20, 40, 50, 75, 100 yards

    (b) Backward—record speed for 5, 10, 15 yards

    (c) Slide Step—record speed for 5, 10, 15 yards

    (d) Carioca—record speed for 5, 10, 15 yards

3. *Endurance Running*

    (a) Forward—440 yards

    (b) Forward—880 yards

    (c) Forward—1 mile

4. *Pattern Running*

    (a) Combine forward, backward, slide step, and carioca running in timed drills over prescribed patterns which include immediate reverses, veres, sharp directional changes, and circles. Use lines, cones, bodies, tires, etc., as markers.

Jumping Skills

1. *Hops*

    (a) Single leg hops—10 yards

    (b) Double leg hops—10 yards

    (c) Alternate single leg hops—10 yards

    (d) Alternate single and double leg hops—10 yards

2. *Jumps for distance*

    (a) Single leg standing long jump

    (b) Double leg standing long jump

    (c) Single leg vertical jump

    (d) Double leg vertical jump

    (e) Running long jump

3. *Elemental gymnastic jumps*

    (a) Tuck jump

    (b) Pike jump

    (c) Straddled toe-touch jump

    (d) Vertical jump with ½ twist

    (e) Vertical jump with full twist

    (f) Vertical jump with 1½ twist

    (g) Vertical jump with two twists

4. *Rope skipping*

    (a) Single leg form jumping

    (b) Single leg speed jumping

    (c) Alternate leg form jumping

    (d) Alternate leg speed jumping

    (e) Double leg form jumping

    (f) Double leg speed jumping

    (g) Combined single and double leg patterns displaying form and speed

Balance Skills

1. *Single Leg Balances*

    (a) Foot to knee—eyes closed—10 second hold

    (b) Front scale—5 seconds

    (c) Side scale—5 seconds

    (d) Rear scale—5 seconds

2. *Elemental Hand and Head Balances*

    (a) Tripod—5 seconds

    (b) Frog stand—5 seconds

    (c) Head stand—5 seconds

    (d) Hand stand—5 seconds

3. *Moving Balances*

    (a) Handstand walk—10 feet

    (b) Simple walk—across 4-inch balance beam

    (c) Single leg hops—across 4-inch balance beam

    (d) Backward walk—across 4-inch balance beam

    (e) Backward single leg hops—across 4-inch balance beam

    (f) Single and double leg hops over a variety of prescribed zig-zag patterns using lines, cones, bodies, ropes, tires, as markers and/or obstacles

Miscellaneous Agility Skills

1. *Hands and Feet Skills*

    (a) Forward "Crab-Crawl" Scramble

    (b) Backward "Crab-Crawl" Scramble

    (c) Forward "Dog-Run" Scramble

    (d) Lateral "Dog-Run" Scramble

    (e) Backward "Dog-Run" Scramble

    (f) Circle running around a one-hand-to-the-ground support

    (g) Circle running around a both-hands-to-the-ground support

2. *Break Downs*

    From a standing position, at command snap to a predetermined "get-set" position. The position may be a basketball defense position or a football lineman's stance or something similar.

3. *Down-Ups*

    From a standing position, at command drop to prone position with chest to ground and immediately return to standing position *or* some prescribed stance

Tumbling Skills

1. *Log rolls, right and left*

2. *Shoulder stand balance*

3. *Shoulder stand to forward roll up to stand*

4. *Shoulder stand; lower feet to floor in back of head; use hands to push body backwards to stand*

5. *Forward roll*

6. *Backward roll*

7. *Back extension through handstand*

8. *Cartwheel, right and left*

9. *Cartwheel series*

10. *From a push-up support position:*

    (a) Double leg squat through to seat

    (b) Double leg stoop through (legs straight) to seat

    (c) Double leg flank vault right to seat

    (d) Double leg flank vault left to seat

    (e) Straddle cut to seat

11. *Headspring with spot*

12. *Front handspring with spot*

13. *Front somersault onto foam crash pad*

Mini-Tramp Skills

1. *Bounce and leap straight body.* Attain maximum height *and* body control. Land on foam crash pad placed next to mini-tramp. Always use the crash pad and always have a person to spot.

2. *Bounce and execute straight body jump with one-half twist*

3. *Bounce and execute straight body jump with full twist*

4. *Bounce and execute tuck jump*

5. *Bounce and execute pike jump*

6. *Bounce and execute straddle jump*

7. *With the assistance of two spotters and a spotting belt, bounce, and execute:*
    a) a high dive roll
    b) a tuck front salto
    c) a pike front salto
    d) a back tuck salto

Trampoline Skills

1. *Hands and Knees Drop*

2. *Knee Drop*

3. *Seat Drop*

4. *Front Drop*

5. *Back Drop*

6. *Seat Drop to Saddle—Cut to Front Drop*

7. *Front Drop to Straddle—Cut to Seat Drop*

8. *Seat Drop to Half-Turn to Seat Drop*

9. *Seat Drop to Full-Turn to Seat Drop*

10. *Back Drop to Half-Turn to Stand*

11. *Combination of basic skills*

12. *Forward and backward somersault progressions using overhead spotting belts*

Selected Gymnastic Apparatus Skills

1. *Climbing Rope*
   - (a) Chins starting from seated position
   - (b) Chins started from hanging position
   - (c) Arms and legs climb—20 feet
   - (d) Arms only climb—20 feet

2. *Horizontal Bar*
   - (a) Hangs and swings using all possible hand grip positions
   - (b) "Skin the cat" hang—full shoulder extension
   - (c) Pullover to support
   - (d) Backward simple hip-circle
   - (e) Forward simple hip-circle
   - (f) Kips

3. *Parallel Bars*
   - (a) From support position, walk the length of bars on hands
   - (b) From support position, hop the length of bars on hands
   - (c) From support position, swing forward to straddle seat
   - (d) From support position, swing backward to straddle seat
   - (e) From support position, execute swing and straddle seats the length of bars. Execute both forward and backward
   - (f) From support position, straight arm—straight body swings, relaxed and controlled
   - (g) From support position, execute swinging dips
   - (h) From support position, execute simple front and rear dismounts
   - (i) Shoulder stand
   - (j) L support
   - (k) Rolls, kips, and uprises

4. *Still Rings*
   (a) "Bird's nest" hang
   (b) "Skin the cat" hang
   (c) Piked hang
   (d) Inverted straight body hang
   (e) Muscle up
   (f) L support
   (g) Shoulder stand
   (h) Kips, forward and backward
   (i) Simple swing
   (j) Dislocates, inlocates, uprises *with spotters*

5. *Side Horse*
   (a) Squat vault
   (b) Straddle vault
   (c) Flank vaults, right and left
   (d) From support, execute single leg cuts right and left
   (e) From support, execute forward scissors right and left
   (f) From support, execute simple travels from end to middle and middle to end

TYPICAL DRILLS FOR QUICKNESS AND AGILITY

Quick Drills

1. *From standing position:*
   (a) Tuck jump; break down; on command sprint 5 yards
   (b) Pike jump; break down; on command sprint 5 yards
   (c) Straddle jump; break down; on command sprint 5 yards
   (d) Jump with full twist; break down; on command sprint 5 yards
   (e) Jump with full twist right, then left; break down, on command sprint 5 yards
   (f) Forward roll; break down; on command sprint 5 yards
   (g) Backward roll; break down; on command sprint 5 yards
   (h) Backward roll; forward roll; break down; on command sprint 5 yards.

(i) Tuck jump; forward roll; break down; on command sprint 5 yards

(j) Pike jump; forward roll; break down; on command sprint 5 yards

(k) Straddle jump; forward roll; break down; on command sprint 5 yards

(l) Full twist right and left; forward roll; break down; on command sprint 5 yards

(m) Full twist right and left; forward roll; tuck jump; break down; on command sprint 5 yards

(n) Full twist right and left; forward roll; pike jump; break down; on command sprint 5 yards

(o) Full twist right and left; forward roll; straddle jump; break down; on command sprint 5 yards

(p) Full twist right and left; backward roll; forward roll; tuck jump; break down; on command sprint 5 yards

(q) Full twist right and left; backward roll; forward roll; straddle jump; break down; on command sprint 5 yards

(r) Full twist right and left; backward roll; forward roll; pike jump; break down; on command sprint 5 yards

(s) Drop to "Dog-Run" scramble position, full circle right, left, snap up and sprint 5 yards

(t) Three-quarter eagle drill—simple break down, on command ¼ turn right, return, ¼ turn left, return, one down up and sprint 5 yards

Agility Drills

1. *Break down and on command:*
   (a) Twisting run for 10 yards; forward sprint for 10 yards
   (b) Backward run for 10 yards; forward sprint for 10 yards
   (c) Carioca run for 10 yards; forward sprint for 10 yards
   (d) One leg hop for 10 yards; forward sprint for 10 yards
   (e) Two leg hop for 10 yards; forward sprint for 10 yards
   (f) "Dog-Run" scramble for 10 yards; forward sprint for 10 yards

(g) Front "Crab-Crawl" for 10 yards; forward sprint for 10 yards

(h) Back "Crab-Crawl" for 10 yards; forward sprint for 10 yards

(i) Forward sprint for 10 yards; circle right around one hand support; forward sprint for 10 yards; circle left around one hand support

2. *Wave Drill*

Following hand signals of instructor, run diagonally right or left changing with signals; 10 yards

3. *Mirror Drill*

Two partners face each other with one designated leader. Object is to mirror the leader for 10 seconds. Encourage a variety of movements.

4. *Backward Running—Break Down—Forward Running*

(a) Backward for 5 yards; forward for 5 yards

(b) Backward for 10 yards; forward for 10 yards

(c) Backward for 15 yards; forward for 15 yards

(d) Backward for 20 yards; forward for 20 yards

5. *Over and Back*

(a) Forward running for 5 yards; turn; forward running to starting point

(b) Forward running for 10 yards; turn; forward running to starting point

(c) Forward running for 15 yards; turn; forward running to starting point

(d) Forward running for 20 yards; turn; forward running to starting point

6. *Human Circles*

Form circle with 10 people lying on stomach, heads to center, hips 1-2 yards apart. Designate a starter. When he passes over the number 2 man, then the number 2 man gets up and begins, and so on until every man in the circle has performed and returned to his starting position. Use the following skills:

(a) Two leg hops

(b) Single leg hops

(c) Sideward running with both feet touching in each space

(d) Forward running with only one foot touching in each space

Use many circles and incorporate relay situations.

7. *Cone Drills*

Place four cones so that they form a square with each side equaling 5 yards.

(a) Starting 1 yard away from cone one (left)

(b) On command place right hand beside cone and circle right

(c) Sprint to cone two and place left hand beside cone; circle left

(d) Sprint to cone three and place left hand beside cone; circle left

(e) Sprint to final cone and place right hand beside cone; circle right; cross finish line

This is an excellent drill for balance, speed acceleration from one point to another, and also quick change of direction. Run this one for time.

CONCLUDING REMARKS

The application of muscle responsiveness exercises combined with concentrated work on the fundamental skills of human movement will develop a total athlete. He will be knowledgeable and have positive attitudes about human movement and also injury prevention. He will acquire suppleness, elasticity, and maximum range of movement. He will attain total body development. His neuromuscular control will improve; his coordination will refine. He will be nimble and light on his feet. His improved balance, equilibrium, and kinesthetic awareness, even in foreign positions, will help promote an increased agility spectrum. The program, kept fresh, exciting, and competitive by a variety of mass drills, will also improve the individual's mental attitudes, including self-discipline, confidence, fearlessness, daring, courage, initiative, decisiveness, determination, and poise.

Part Three

Team Drills

6

Team Warmup Program

The goals of a good team warmup program are the following:

1. To begin each practice with a good team atmosphere.

2. To provide a series of exercises designed to increase circulation, stretch the muscles, improve freedom of motion, and prepare the body for the more vigorous exercise demands of the practice session.

3. To develop and improve flexibility progressively.

4. To reduce as much as possible the athlete's potential for pulls and strains.

5. To improve muscular relaxation.

6. To improve muscle quickness for better change of direction capability.

7. To improve self-awareness of muscle needs.

8. To provide a daily program of football flexibility needs.

PROCEDURE

The team assembles as a group in exercise formation. The attitude should be relaxed but attentive and serious—quiet concentration is preferable for best results. The exercises should be performed in the same manner, direction, and pace as the coach or leader. Always do the best you can, but never force an exercise. Permit the benefits of the exercise to occur in a progressive manner.

When exercises are concluded, the team breaks and goes to individual coaches.

WARMUP PROGRAM

Exercise 1. *Running in Place*

Running in place stimulates the circulation to open up the capillary network and aids in both the performance and benefits of the flexibility exercises. Duration of this exercise should be at least 20 seconds. Alternatives which may be used on occasion include jumping jacks, rope skipping, or a ¼-mile jog.

Exercise 2. *Relaxed Bouncing in Place*

Perform 10 simple bounces on the balls of the feet. Relax as much as possible, breathing easily. Begin now to pay complete attention to proper performance of the exercises and also the way your muscles respond. Circulation, relaxation, and concentration help you derive maximum benefits from the program.

Exercise 3. *Fingers and Wrists*

1. Interlock fingers and press palms together.

2. Using pressure, rotate the wrists in a variety of directions.

3. Keep fingers interlocked.

4. Turn thumbs down and palms away from body. Straighten the arms forward then overhead.

5. Press palms together.

6. Press backs of hands together.

Exercise 4. *Elbow Flexion and Extension*

Using pressure, flex and extend each elbow. This is a very simple exercise and you may feel nothing. However, if any irritation is present, this exercise will probably reveal it and indicate that you should spend extra time later warming up this area.

Exercise 5. *Arm Circles and Swings*

Relaxed swinging of the arms in the following ways:

(a) 10 arm circles forward.

(b) 10 arm circles backward.

(c) 10 over-and-under horizontal arm swings with lateral trunk twist.

(d) 10 cross-and-swing horizontal arm swings with lateral trunk twist.

Exercise 6. *Neck Circles and Related Movements*

Perform the following:

(a) Rotate the neck 5 times in each direction using fully extended circles.

(b) Move the head from side to side 5 times.

(c) Move the head forward and backward 5 times.

Exercise 7. *Side Bends and Hip Circles*

From straddle stand, perform the following:

(a) 5 side bends to each side, alternating sides.

(b) Perform 5 hip circles in each direction.

Exercise 8. *Stretches from Straddle Stand*

From a wide straddle stand, perform the following:

(a) Reach down the right and hold 5 seconds.

(b) Reach down the left and hold 5 seconds.

(c) Reach down the middle and hold 5 seconds.

(d) Repeat.

Do not bounce. Keep legs straight as possible.

Exercise 9. *Stoop Stand and Pike Stand*

From straight stand, perform the following:

(a) Stoop stand, hands touching the ground. Hold 5 seconds.

(b) Pike stand, hands behind knees. Hold 5 seconds.

Exercise 10. *Squat Stand*

Lower to squat stand with knees bent and hands on the ground. Hold 3 seconds.

Exercise 11. *Arch and Round the Back*

From the hands-and-knees position, arch the back and look up. Next, round the back and look at the knees. Keep the arms straight at all times. Repeat each position 3 times.

Exercise 12. *Knee Scales*

From hands-and-knees, arch the back and lift the right leg as high as possible. Next, bend the knee and swing the leg forward while rounding the back until the knee touches the chest. Repeat 3 times. Repeat procedure with left leg.

Exercise 13. *Arch Rise Combinations*

From hands-and-knees, push back to knee-and-forehead position. Perform the following:

(a) Pull forward to arch rise, push back to knee-and-forehead position. Repeat 3 times, slowly.

(b) From arch rise, lower to on-your-front and push back up to arch rise. Repeat 3 times.

(c) From arch rise, bend knees and hold for 3 seconds.

Exercise 14. *Cradle-Set and Cradle*

From on-your-front, reach back and grab the ankles. Try to touch heels to rear. Next, lift legs and arch body as much as possible. Hold 3 seconds.

Exercise 15. *Ankles*

From straight sit, perform the following:

(a) Rotate the right ankle 5 times in one direction.

(b) Rotate the right ankle 5 times in the other direction.

(c) Flex the right ankle and extend it forcefully against resistance supplied by your hands.

(d) Extend the right ankle and flex it forcefully against resistance supplied by your hands.

(e) Repeat the above steps with the left ankle.

Exercise 16. *Tuck Sits, Single and Double Leg*

From straight sit, perform the following:

(a) Single leg tuck sit right. Hold 2 seconds.

(b) Single leg tuck sit left. Hold 2 seconds.

(c) Double leg tuck sit. Hold 2 seconds.

Exercise 17. *Pike Sits*

From straight sit, perform the following:

(a) Pike sit with ankles extended. Hold 5 seconds.

(b) Pike sit with ankles flexed. Hold 5 seconds.

In each exercise keep the legs straight and do not bounce.

Exercise 18. *Single Leg Lifts from Straight Sit*

From straight sit, perform the following:

(a) Single leg lift right. Hold 5 seconds.

(b) Single leg lift left. Hold 5 seconds.

Keep the legs straight and do not bounce.

Exercise 19. *Single Leg Lifts from Straight-on-Your-Back*

From straight-on-your-back, perform the following:

(a) Single leg lift right. Hold 5 seconds.

(b) Single leg lift left. Hold 5 seconds.

Keep the legs straight and do not bounce.

Exercise 20. *Half Pike Cross-Overs; Deep Pike and Deep Straddle*

From straight-on-the-back, perform the following:

(a) Double leg lift to half pike. Cross and touch the right hand and hold 2 seconds. Cross and touch the left hand and hold 2 seconds.

(b) Deep pike touching toes to the ground. Hands *may* grasp legs to pull the pike tighter.

(c) Deep straddle touching toes to the ground. Hands *may* grasp ankles to pull the straddle deeper.

Exercise 21. *Tuck Straddle Sit*

From tuck sit, straddle the knees and press them to the

ground. Using the arms to supply resistance, press the knees together, then apart, 3 times. Next, grasp the ankles and pull the forehead to the ankles. Hold 3 seconds.

Exercise 22. *Stretches from Straddle Sit*

From straddle sit, perform the following:

(a) Reach down the right leg. Hold 5 seconds.
(b) Reach down the left leg. Hold 5 seconds.
(c) Reach down the middle. Hold 5 seconds.

Keep the legs straight and do not bounce.

Exercise 23. *Stretches from Hurdler's Sit*

Straddle sit with right leg straight, left leg bent, left ankle extended with top of left foot on ground. From the hurdler's sit, perform the following:

(a) Reach down the right. Hold 5 seconds.
(b) Reach down the middle. Hold 5 seconds.
(c) Reach down the left. Hold 5 seconds.
(d) Lie back. Hold 5 seconds.
(e) Repeat from hurdler's sit left.

Exercise 24. *Knee Stand, Quad Stretch*

From knee stand, perform the following:

(a) Lean back ¼. Hold 2 seconds.
(b) Lean back ½. Hold 2 seconds.
(c) Lean back ¾. Hold 2 seconds.
(d) Lean back and touch the ground. Hold 2 seconds.

Exercise 25. *Straddle Lunges*

From straddle stand, perform the following:

(a) Straddle lunge right. Hold 5 seconds.
(b) Straddle lunge left. Hold 5 seconds.
(c) Repeat each.

Do not bounce.

Exercise 26. *Split Lunges*

From straddle stand, perform the following:

(a) Split lunge right. Hold 5 seconds.

(b) Split lunge left. Hold 5 seconds.

(c) Repeat each.

Do not bounce.

Exercise 27. *Splits*

Perform the following:

(a) Split right. Use hands for support. Hold 5 seconds.

(b) Split left. Use hands for support. Hold 5 seconds.

(c) Wide straddle split. Hold 5 seconds.

Do not bounce. Do each exercise the best you can. Do not force.

Exercise 28. *Single and Double Arm Shoulder Stretches*

From straight sit, perform the following:

(a) Reach back as far as possible with the right arm. Hold 3 seconds.

(b) Reach back as far as possible with the left arm. Hold 3 seconds.

(c) Reach back as far as possible with both arms. Hold 3 seconds.

Exercise 29. *Rock Back and Rock Forward*

From tuck sit, grasp the knees and rock back and forward 3 times.

Exercise 30. *Squat Straddle Stand*

From squat straddle stand, perform the following:

(a) Press the knees together against resistance supplied by arms.

(b) Press the legs apart against resistance supplied by arms.

(c) Repeat each 3 times.

Exercise 31. *Balance Drill*

From straight stand, perform the following:

(a) Lift the right leg forward, then to the side, and finally to the back. Control your balance through the entire sequence.

(b) Repeat with the left leg.

Exercise 32. *Inlocates and Dislocates*

1. Grasp the wand or exertube in overgrip and perform the following:

(a) Raise wand or tube overhead and inlocate (let the shoulders roll).

(b) Touch the wand or tube to your rear, then bring it forward and dislocate.

(c) Repeat 10 times, slowly.

2. Grasp the wand or exertube in undergrip and perform the following:

(a) Raise the wand from your rear overhead and dislocate (let the shoulders roll).

(b) Lower the wand or tube forward to touch your legs. Keep the palms forward.

(c) Reverse the procedure; inlocate.

(d) Repeat 10 times, slowly.

Exercise 33. *Running in Place*

Conclude the warmup as it started, running in place for 20 seconds or jumping jacks, rope skipping, a ¼-mile run, or agility drills including forward and backward running, and carioca running.

RAINDAY WARMUP PROGRAM

On inclement weather days, do exercises 1-8 of the Team Warmup Program and add the following exercise.

Straddle Lunges

From straddle stand, perform the following:

(a) Straddle lunge right. Hold 5 seconds.

(b) Straddle lunge left. Hold 5 seconds.

(c) Repeat both.

Do not bounce.

7

Team Warmdown Program

Warmdowns are designed to use body heat, increased circulation, and flexibility exercises to cleanse fatigue products, relax and stretch muscles, and reduce soreness.

The goals of a good team warmdown program are:

1. To conclude each practice with a good team atmosphere.

2. To provide a short series of exercises designed to maintain a slight circulation increase, stretch the muscles, relax the muscles, and permit some cleansing of waste products.

3. To serve as an additional effort to improve flexibility.

4. To serve as an additional effort to reduce the athlete's potential for pulls and strains.

5. To aid in reducing muscle soreness.

6. To improve self-awareness of muscle needs.

7. To provide a daily program of post-practice needs in the areas of flexibility, muscle relaxation, waste product removal, and injury reduction.

Procedure

The team assembles as a group or in groups by position. The attitude should be relaxed and attentive—quiet concentration is preferable for best results. The exercises should be performed in the same manner as the coach or leader.

Always do your best, but never force an exercise. Permit the benefits of the exercise to occur in a progressive manner. When exercises are concluded, practice is over.

Exercise 1. *Squat Stand*

Lower to squat stand with knees bent and hands on the ground. Hold 3 seconds.

Exercise 2. *Squat Straddle Stand*

From squat straddle stand, perform the following:

(a) Press the knees together against resistance supplied by arms.

(b) Press the legs apart against resistance supplied by arms.

(c) Repeat each 3 times.

Exercise 3. *Stretches from Straddle Sit*

From straddle sit, perform the following:

(a) Reach down the right leg. Hold 5 seconds.

(b) Reach down the left leg. Hold 5 seconds.

(c) Reach down the middle. Hold 5 seconds.

Keep the legs straight and do not bounce.

Exercise 4. *Stretches from Hurdler's Sit*

Straddle sit with right leg straight, left leg bent, left ankle extended with top of left foot on ground. From the hurdler's sit, perform the following:

(a) Reach down the right. Hold 5 seconds.

(b) Reach down the middle. Hold 5 seconds.

(c) Reach down the left. Hold 5 seconds.

(d) Lie back. Hold 5 seconds.

(e) Repeat from hurdler's sit left.

Exercise 5. *Knee Stand, Quad Stretch*

From knee stand, perform the following:

(a) Lean back ¼. Hold 2 seconds.
(b) Lean back ½. Hold 2 seconds.
(c) Lean back ¾. Hold 2 seconds.
(d) Lean back and touch the ground. Hold 2 seconds.

Exercise 6. *Straddle Lunges*

From straddle stand, perform the following:

(a) Straddle lunge right. Hold 5 seconds.
(b) Straddle lunge left. Hold 5 seconds.
(c) Repeat each.

Do not bounce.

Exercise 7. *Split Lunges*

From straddle stand, perform the following:

(a) Make ¼ turn and split lunge right. Hold 5 seconds.
(b) Make ½ turn and split lunge left. Hold 5 seconds.
(c) Repeat each.

Do not bounce.

Exercise 8. *Stretches from Straddle Stand*

From a wide straddle stand, perform the following:

(a) Reach down the right and hold 5 seconds.
(b) Reach down the left and hold 5 seconds.
(c) Reach down the middle and hold 5 seconds.
(d) Repeat.

Do not bounce. Keep legs straight as possible.

Exercise 9. *Stoop Stand and Pike Stand*

From straight stand, perform the following:

(a) Stoop stand, hands touching the ground. Hold 5 seconds.
(b) Pike stand, hands behind knees. Hold 5 seconds.

8

Outlining A Training Program

Here is an outline of a training program for a professional football player, including pre-season, training camp, season, and post season sessions. Use this as a guideline in formulating your own personal long-term workouts. Your outline will obviously be different and highly individualized to suit your personal athletic needs. The important point is to plan ahead, state general and specific objectives, and then follow your planning as close as possible.

WEEK 1

Morning Training (20-30 minutes)

Jog, warmup program, and selected stretching, 3-minute run at moderate pace, warmdown.

Afternoon Program (1 hour)

Jog, warmup, agility drills, extensive flexibility workout, one-mile run, warmdown.

WEEK 2

Morning Training (20-30 minutes)

Afternoon Program (1 hour)

Jog, warmup, agility drills, partner-assisted resistive flexibility program, strength program, one-mile run, warmdown.

WEEK 3

Morning Training (20-30 minutes)

Afternoon Program (1 hour, 20 minutes)

Jog, warmup, agility drills, flexibility, strength, and speed workout, one-mile run, warmdown.

WEEK 4

Morning Training (20-30 minutes)

Afternoon Program (1 hour, 30 minutes)

Flexibility program and endurance program, and 12-minute run and warmdown; Tuesday, Thursday, Saturday—same as week 3.

WEEK 5

Morning Training (20-30 minutes)

Afternoon Program (1 hour, 30 minutes)

Monday and Wednesday:	Flexibility, endurance, 12-minute run, and warmdown.
Tuesday:	Flexibility, strength, agility, sports skills, and warmdown.
Thursday:	Flexibility, strength, speed, sports skills, and warmdown.
Friday and Saturday:	Flexibility, speed, sports skills, and warmdown.

WEEK 6

Morning Training (20-30 minutes)

Afternoon Program (1 hour, 30 minutes)

Monday: Flexibility, strength, speed, agilities, and warm-down.

Tuesday: Flexibility, sports skills, endurance, and warm-down.

Wednesday: Flexibility, speed, agilities, sports skills, and warmdown.

Thursday: Flexibility, strength, 12-minute run, and warm-down.

Friday: Flexibility, endurance, and warmdown.

Saturday: Flexibilty, sports skills, agilities, 12-minute run, and warmdown.

TRAINING CAMP

Morning Training (10-15 minutes)

Warmup and warmdown after each practice.

Monday, Wednesday,
and Friday: Strength workout

Tuesday and Thursday: Endurance workout

Saturday: 12-minute run, or selected intense football running drills (12 minutes)

SEASON

Monday: Rest
Tuesday: Flexibility session and strength
Wednesday: Flexibility session and 4-minute run
Thursday: Flexibility session and strength
Friday: Flexibility session and 2-minute run
Saturday: Flexibility session

OFF-SEASON

First Six Weeks

Rest and flexibility exercise only.

Second Six Weeks

Flexibility, strength, and speed.

Flexibility: every day

Strength: three days per week

Speed: three days per week

Repeat six weeks pre-season training to prepare for camp.

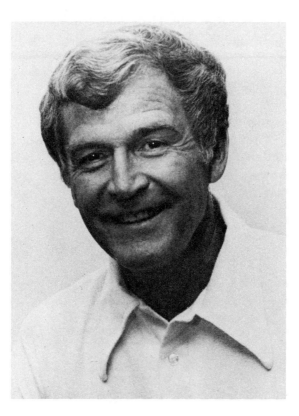

About the Author

Paul Uram recently retired his position as an assistant coach with the Pittsburgh Steelers. He has also coached with the Washington Redskins and the Baltimore Colts, each in the year they went to the Super Bowl. Part of the credit for the success of teams Uram has worked with must go to his conditioning program, known as Refining Human Movement, which dramatically reduces certain types of injuries.

The Refining Human Movement Program is valuable for more than injury prevention. Professional golfers, baseball players, and track stars have sought Uram's help in improving their strength and agility. In all, Uram has consulted with ten

NFL teams and scores of professional and college baseball, basketball, track, and gymnastics teams. The past decade has seen virtually all major sports teams discard conventional calisthenics in favor of a conditioning program modeled after Refining Human Movement.

Uram is a native of Butler, Pennsylvania, where he coached the gymnastics team to a 107-0 record. He received a master's degree in Physical Education from Slippery Rock College, where he lettered in football and track.

He is now devoting his time to teaching, writing and lecturing.